PROVIDING AFFORDABLE, QUALITY HEALTH CARE IN OWERRI:

A Case Study Of The Health Care System In Nigeria

by

Lambert C. Nwachukwu

A Dissertation Presented in Partial Fulfillment

Of the Requirements for the Degree

Professional Doctorate of Business Administration (DBA)

in

Healthcare Management, Leadership, and Public Policy

California Intercontinental University

February 2014

Order this book online at www.trafford.com
or email orders@trafford.com

Most Trafford titles are also available at major online book retailers.

Printed in the United States of America.

ISBN: 978-1-4907-4945-7 (sc)
        978-1-4907-4944-0 (e)

Trafford rev. 11/14/2014

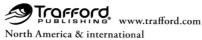 www.trafford.com

North America & international
toll-free: 1 888 232 4444 (USA & Canada)
fax: 812 355 4082

Abstract

Writing on behalf of a community regarding their medical needs and demands offers the chance to avail the community to modern health care services. However, in the city of Owerri located within the state of Imo, obtaining quality medical services remains difficult. The main research question explored the delivery of health care within Owerri. Service delivery models, multi-level governance, and a generalized theory of organized change framed the study. Participants were selected from several educational and professional institutions throughout Owerri. Data was analyzed using open coding strategies and comparative descriptive statistics. Triangulation was ensured by the use of an extensive surveying instrument able to verify the consistency of responses. The results included many recommendations involving governance, individuals, and technology as to create the needed infrastructure allowing delivery of medical services matching the demand within the borders of Owerri. Although the results may not be generalizable beyond the region of the study, its findings may support sound policies aiming to provide effective health care services to those who need it within Owerri and similar contexts within Nigeria.

Dedication

I dedicate this work to my mother who instilled the quest, love and thirst for education at an early stage as a child. I also dedicate this day to my wife who encouraged and supported my going to graduate school without which this would not have been possible. Above all, I dedicate the completion of this project to God Almighty, to which this achievement and all Glory shall always be.

Acknowledgements

I owe the completion of this work to my advisor and supervisor, Prof. Troy Roland; who encouraged, advised and directed me in this project. My special thanks to Dr. Andrea Clarke of the student services for her support and encouragement. My warmest greetings to Terry Ruiz of the admissions department for her admission support for sticking around with me and insisting and reminding me about the affordability at CalU—*The CalU Advantage*. Most importantly my appreciation to CalU for the tuition payment plan without which this would have not been possible. I also acknowledge and appreciate the effort of my younger brother, Mr. Reginald Nwachukwu for his diligent effort in executing and coordinating the questionnaires. Thanks to all my wonderfully exceptional friends and those I met at CalU for their help, and encouragement for their pieces of advice. I also thank Dr. Peter Nanopoulos for his guidance and wonderful support in the production of this document. The completion of this document is and will continue to be an accomplishment and a big step forward in the overall achievement and success in my life. It is also a brave distinction in the academic pursuit and destination of my life and the academic conquest.

Steven Hess, PhD, Chair

Amarjit Singh, PhD, Committee Member

Andrea Clarke, DBA, Committee Member

Table of Contents

Table of Figures

Chapter 1: Introduction

Leaders and those aspiring to direct the welfare of a nation need to understand how citizens perceive the institutions of nation. When the publicly sponsored institution administering the welfare of a nation via health care policies falls into crisis, its leaders must understand the nature of the crisis and influence upon the health of citizens. The adage, reality is perception remains true during such a crisis as leaders ask how to coordinate the resources of a nation as to address a health crisis. This study frames a crisis of health care services delivery within the city of Owerri located within the state of Imo, Nigeria. The goal of this study is to richly illustrate and research the failure of government institutions within Owerri as to understand the problems facing the Nigerian health care sector.

Background of the Problem

This study sought to identify, describe, and analyze the state of health care in Nigeria, with primary research focus placed upon the city of Owerri and in the wider geographic area of Imo State. A brief historical background of the evolution of health care policy in Nigeria in an effort to explain current needs, and to describe these needs by using primary and secondary empirical data. A preliminary yet diligent review of the literature reveals some missing gaps in the development and delivery of health care services, and this study is designed to explore the reasons for these gaps and to propose actionable policy recommendations to local and national governments. An additional component of the paper explored the concept of rural infrastructural development in Nigeria as a foundation to current healthcare crisis. Thus, exploring the direction and extent to which this lead to the Owerri healthcare issues and gaps becomes a major focus.

Infrastructure Development Prior to 1945

Public or governmental involvement in infrastructural development dates to approximately 1917 when the colonial government promulgated township ordinances. Ordinances established three kinds of settlements: (a) First Class Townships; (b) Second Class Townships; and (c) Third Class Townships. First Class Townships, such as Lagos, held a White population and workforce resting upon a heavy concentration of infrastructure and services (Olayiwola and Adeleye, 2005). Conversely, Second and Third Class Townships contained little or no infrastructure until the 1952. The authors believed that the establishment of the Local Government Councils in Western Nigeria in 1952 sought to extend infrastructure into rural areas. Unfortunately, the allocated funding to local governments as to pay for infrastructure expansion barely funded the council headquarters and health care services (Olayiwola et al, 2005). Little or no funding remained to initiate new schemes for rural development.

Infrastructure Development from 1945 to 2008

Ajovi and Scott-Emuakpor (2010) characterize the evolution of health care services in Nigeria as a sequence of short term planning strategies mimicking most aspects of Nigerian life. The evolutions, illustrated as a succession of National Development Plans, formulated goals for nationwide health care services. Since urban services were well developed during the lifetime of the Plans, government planners intended to develop health service within rural areas. Such services would appear as rural hospitals containing approximately two dozen beds, supervised medical officers and dispensaries, welfare clinics, and preventive work projects including sanitation services. The Plans required sharing the costs of development between regional and national governments via grants and local funding. Although the Plans remained ambitious and wanting to develop rural infrastructure, General Yakubu Gowon stated, "Development trends in the health sector have not been marked by any spectacular achievement during the past decade." Thus despite the vision of the plans, very little development occurred while improving the numerical strength of existing facilities - rather than evolving a clear health care policy.

The Establishment of Health Care

The development of health care delivery services backed by public education campaigns can prevent unnecessary death and suffering in rural areas. For example, many childhood illnesses such as polio, measles, and mumps, may be prevented using basic health services and vaccinations. The effectiveness of such programs are reflected in the recent near eradication of polio from Nigeria. Thus, the establishment of health care services can affect maternal mortality, mosquito larvae risks, health sector reform, and the financing of health care ventures.

Maternal Mortality. Maternal mortality is a cause of concern because most pregnant women lack access to prenatal and postnatal care (Scott-Ememuakpor, 2010). WHO (2010) defines maternal maternity rate (MMR) as death of women while pregnant or within 42 days after termination of pregnancy irrespective of duration or site of pregnancy. This is a global challenge particularly in the continent of Africa. According WHO, among the countries examined and surveyed, Nigeria ranked 11th with a death rate of 630/100,000 births.

Mosquito larvae education. In Owerri, as in other parts of Nigeria, malaria is a preventable and prevalent cause of death. The lack of infrastructure, public education, and delivery of drugs such as Pyrimethamine, Chloroquine, and Artesunate coupled to use of the barrier method, hamper efforts aiming to reduce the spread of malaria. Thus developing related infrastructure and health care delivery services may improve public health, reduce the occurrences of standing water acting as incubators for mosquito larvae, and establish preventive practices. In turn, people live healthier lives and government benefits by a reduction in the days lost by workers due to preventable diseases.

Recent health sector reforms. Recent reforms focused upon establishing a national health policy in Nigeria demands the existence of a responsive and effective health system based upon primary health care enabling all citizens to live socially and economically productive lives (DFID, 2000). According to Saka and Asuzu (2007), the public debate over health care reform in Nigeria is driven by a wide variety of policy issues, including the role of the local administrative bodies and the duties of the state authorities. Despite debates and the focus of reforms, the Nigerian citizen has only the testimony of words and not the actions leading to reform. Although the debates place policy makers and policies in the limelight, policy makers tend to ignore the commitment of citizens in establishing affordable quality health care services delivery.

Financing concerns. Although undocumented, it is commonly accepted that the Nigerian health care system remains underdeveloped, mismanaged, and unable to meet the demands placed upon it. The World Health Organization reported Nigeria had the highest drug prices in the world coupled to a statistic indicating citizens often spend 23% of their income on medicine (Megagji, 2010; Mourik et al., 2010; WHO, 2000).

Additionally, Ogundipe (2010) observed that the average drug price in Nigeria is 82% higher than the next country in a group of eight nations with the highest drug prices in the world. The recent study performed by Ammon (2008) illustrated the Nigerian marketplace as one of the few countries in the world with a high prevalence of counterfeit drugs. Such indicators reflect a health care system lacking capital investment (Garuba, Kohler, & Huisman, 2009).

The lack of capital investment undermines the capacity of firms to fund research and development efforts because of the high costs of procuring materials and technologies compliant with WHO standards (Erhum et al., 2001; Okhamefe, 2006). Although it is a simple matter to equivocate funding with infrastructure, it remains difficult to determine the magnitude and proper implementation of capital investment within the Nigerian health services sector. The difficulty in determination appears to be rooted in the informally discussed culture of corruption practiced by business leaders and elected officials involved with the health delivery industry. Such a culture leads to enhanced investment risk, default concerns, and currency exchange rates making investment into health delivery ventures less attractive to potential investors.

Summary

Despite the well intentioned reform efforts of the last 20 years, the Nigerian health care remains stalled by political and economic stagnation, ineffective coordination of resources, lack of investment capital, poor public education regarding medical options, unaddressed demands upon the health care services sector, and insufficient infrastructure planning. The culmination of these factors leads to the currently observed current healthcare crisis both at the national and local levels within Nigeria. Further, such problems are not strictly the forces, but also result from a disregard for social welfare grounded in corruptive practices, lack of personal responsibility, and poor administrative oversight of the health care services sector.

Problem Statement

There is a problem in the town of Owerri, Nigeria. Despite intense individual efforts to combat unacceptable infant mortality rates, the spread of HIV and AIDS, the effects of insufficient infrastructure, and lack of emergency medical services, there does not yet exist actionable information or polices as to address such problems (Ajovi & Scott-Emuakpor, 2010). This problem negatively affects residents of Owerri because the lack of actionable information denies the chance for its residence to access properly administered health care programs. The problem, rooted in social upheavals, political conflicts, corruptive practices, and the unwillingness of previous governments to provide for the residence of Owerri drives the current manifestation of the problem (Ajovi & Scott-Emuakpor, 2010). Perhaps a study, which investigates the lack of actionable information using a mixed methods methodology and literature review, could provide a solution.

Purpose of the Study

The purpose of this mixed methods methodology was to analyze healthcare service delivery at Owerri for adults involved with the Federal Medical Center of Owerri (FMCO), the Community Health Center in Owerri (CHCO), Imo State University (IMSU), Federal University of Technology, Owerri (FUTO) and Alvan Ikoku College of Education, Owerri. Data was obtained through questionnaires, interviews relevant case studies, policy reports, and similar dissertations and managed using interview memos, anonymized survey outcomes, and literature review notes.

Significance of the Study

The significance of the study resided in its potential to illustrate the health care service delivery needs of Owerri while revealing the challenges facing the implementation of health care delivery in the region. Further, the review of the scarce literature and survey data provided the insight needed by policy makers as to improve the healthcare sector at local and national levels. Such improvements may manifest as the development of training and education for the healthcare organizations, their workers, and health orientated institutions serving Owerri. Thus the ultimate significance of the study, although beyond the scope of this research project, remained with the ability for the data and recommendations to motivate the establishment of efficient, affordable, and effective health care services at the local, regional, and national levels.

Conceptual Framework

Before continuing this work, it is advisable to create and briefly review the conceptual framework in this project to better understand and review the background of the project further. The models employed and applied by the researcher in this document have been studied and applied by previous researchers under different contexts. These frameworks are embraced because of their importance and related to the Owerri experience as to help understand and give more in-depth meaning to the situation. These are presented under the following factors:

Factor 1: The Service Delivery Model:

As noted by UNDP (199o), this model talks about proficiency or efficiency and excellence in the public service delivery system such as healthcare particularly the rural areas. The model tries to explain and sorts the best mechanism to serve, supply, and deliver the product to the people such as Owerri and their healthcare issues.

Factor 2: The Multi-Level Governance Model:

Stubbs (2005) defines this model as a system of government model that promotes neo-pluralism, meaning recognizing the presence and participation of different networks and political communities in the decision - making process outside the interested parties. This is important to the Owerri case where the public and private parties are incorporated in the decision-making process. It also suggests a wide array of determinants that influence the decision of consumers (such as the Owerri people) in seeking healthcare service including the sharing of powers and administrative oversight.

Factor 3: The Medical Choice-Making Model

This is a psychological concept model proposed by Young (1981) showing how personal perceptual factors influence healthcare service choice decision-making processes applicable to the context of Owerri. It also tries to evaluate the culture, knowledge, belief and other perceptions that can prevent or influence the accessibility of healthcare as it relates to customers such as the city of Owerri by paying attention to the role of medical treatment choice options.

Factor 4: The Rural Infrastructure Model

According to Abumere (2002), this model upholds the importance and effectiveness of the development and supply of rural infrastructure as a means of improving the overall quality of life for the local population such as Owerri as a system usually adopted by developing countries such as Nigeria for public service delivery. The model believes that for public service delivery to succeed and extend to local areas, adequate infrastructure facilities must be provided and supported by an efficient, sustainable management and other administrative mechanisms installed to eliminate corruption and potential problems hampering or constraining local progress.

Factor 5: The Theory of Organizational Change

As noted by Cummings & Worley (2005), this theory is employed in this research project because is necessary for people to achieve their objectives without constraints. The key to this model stems from the fact that it believes that change is necessary to change the status quo (as in Owerri healthcare sector), and is more effective and successful when the change is inspired and comes from within, and planned with increasing pressure to those forces pushing change, which produces a higher level of performance in the process.

Building the Model

In this research, the researcher has articulated these models in the conceptual framework that highlights the approaches used to explain the fundamental needs for change in the Owerri healthcare service sector. This articulation helps to buttress the research work in support to accomplishing its objectives in the context. It also incorporates and shows how those factors responsible for change can be modified in other to achieve the target transformation becomes the focal point in the discussion.

Research Questions

The research questions that guided this study were:

Research Question 1: How can health care delivery in Owerri be modified as to meet market and social demands?

Research Question 2: What kinds of policy recommendations may help alleviate the problem of care delivery in Owerri?

Assumptions, Limitations, and Delimitations

This study assumed the concerns surrounding the use of a survey involving a difficult to access sample and limited literature requiring a narrow scope of inquiry. Further, the limitations and delimitations of the study reflected this fact while demanding a tight focus upon a targeted group of participants.

Assumptions

The sparse nature of the literature requires the study to assume the validity and measures derived from the survey instrument. Thus the study assumes that participants will answer the questionnaires honestly and truthful to best of their ability without fear of punishment. Such an assumption is justified because participants are volunteers able to excuse themselves from the survey. The study further assumes the sample represents the population of Owerri.

Limitations

The study faced naturally occurring limitation concerning time, data collection, and sample size. Data collection and sample size concerns emerged as naturally occurring limitations because it was difficult to establish a large survey group with knowledge of health services in Owerri. The survey also faced limitations involving the perception of employer retribution given participation in the survey process. Although such limitations constrain the generalizability of the survey, they were considered as acceptable due to the difficulties faced when surveying such a specialized pool of participants.

Delimitations

The study contained the following delimitations: (a) a selective process in choosing survey questions; (b) the interpretation of data using particular theoretical perspectives appearing within the lens of the study; (c) the geographical area involved with the study; and (d) the use of a narrow problem allowing tractable analysis. Although delimitations may call into question the validity and consistency of the study, they were required as to keep the study focused and appropriate for a small research project.

Definition of Terms

Access. The term describing the ability to utilize healthcare facilities and systems.

Cosmopolitan Networks. Wolinsky (1998b) defines such networks as a collection of people who are open minded, not limited to a circle of friends, or prevented from receiving and using information from other people and sectors.

Culture. The shared behavior and beliefs characteristic of a particular social, ethnic, or age group.

Lay Referral. Cockerham (1982) defines this as a method by which family members or friends can help a sick individual understand the nature of a disease, its symptoms, and treatment options.

Parochial Networks. Wolinsky (1988b) defines this as a social friendship unwilling to accept new ideas or information while sorting out difficult problems associated with illness or interpreting sickness.

Social Networks. Cockerham (1982) defines such networks as a collection of trustworthy individuals able to exchange viewpoints and share ideas.

FRN. Federal Republic of Nigeria

GDP. Gross Domestic Product

DFID. Directorate for International Development

FCT. Federal Capital Territory

FMOH. Federal Ministry of Health

GNP. Gross National Product

NEEDS. National Economic Empowerment and Development Strategy

OOPS. Out of Pocket Spending

PHC. Primary Health Care

WB. World Bank

NGO. Non-Governmental Organization

NNHIS. Nigeria National Health Insurance Scheme

NHS: National Health System

ILO. International Labor Organization

IMF. International Monetary Fund

RUDO. Rural Urban Disparity/Owerri)

SEEDS. IMO State Economic Empowerment and Development Strategy

WHO. World Health Organization

Conclusion

This chapter presented broad view of the problems appearing within the healthcare sector in Nigeria while focusing upon the city of Owerri. This chapter also included an outline and history of health care within the Owerri community. An in depth review of the literature follows in chapter 2, which will expound upon the development and significance of the study and its literature. Chapter 3 includes a discussion on the methodology of the data collected. In Chapter 4, the results and analysis of the study will be presented. Finally, chapter 5 consists of commenting on the study combined with suggestions for future studies stemming from this research.

Chapter 2: Literature Review

Historical Overview of the Problem

In general terms, local or rural societies in Nigeria live in simple traditional and cultural environments. Accordingly, people's living conditions and social relationships or associations including other modes of behavior differ from one local place to another or from one area to another and even from one region of the country to another. These design differences are very much influenced by change. Nigeria is no difference to this type of experience. The understanding and learning of local communities have drawn attention notably in developing economies (such as Nigeria) but also in many other disciplines as healthcare. The unequal and unusual status, the unfortunate dispossessions of the healthcare issues surrounding the area and its occurrences affecting Owerri and its local population, hence prompted this study. Therefore, the healthcare service inequality is one major issue confronting the Owerri population and other local areas in Nigeria. This study is focused on the process of finding ways to solving and alleviating this problem as it relates to Owerri and affects the state of Imo and Nigeria as a whole.

Therefore, the aim of this chapter is to provide a review of selected reports that will be used to give clarity and focus on the research problem. This literature review will examine and focus on Local Government health Service delivery in global, Africa, including Nigeria with particular reference to south and southeastern Nigerian context that are published. Some other works like the impact of decentralization and devolution on Local Government service delivery have also been reviewed in the process in this chapter. The theoretical frame work is addressed mainly with decentralization and multi-level governance models, specifically their meaning, types, dimension, various forms, advantages and disadvantages which they may have in relation to the subject matter. Thus, why decentralization to service delivery and what variables affect the better health care service delivery are discussed. The main issue here is whether or not decentralization has had a positive influence on better healthcare offered and given to the people as well as its utilization in Owerri becomes the focal point.

Critique of the Previous Scholarly Research

In this study, a number of relevant journal articles, reports, and official documents have been consulted and reviewed for the purpose of this study. An attempt has been made to review the papers consulted during the course of the study with particular focus on LG service delivery in Nigeria, Africa and globally. Some other issues like the impact of decentralization and devolution on local government (LG) Service delivery have also been addressed while reviewing the available documents in this research study.

Kamiljon and Felix Asante in their study (2009) deconcentration of community work performance in Ghana: "Do Geography and Ethnic Diversity Matter" published in 2009, tries to explore variations in rural service supply arrangements for the local people of Ghana and the home group quantitative information. According to these authors, localities in a region may play a big role in determining variations in providing access and rendering service to the rural people of Ghana. In this paper, the authors showed that people of different groups have different needs that may influence access and determine the approach to service in fulfilling those needs such as drinking water and power supply, etc. They believe there is a prominent division of people and their needs (services) in these areas that affects how the different groups can use the available services such as pipe borne water in satisfying their need. They also indicated that the demand and division for service decreases as the amount or rate of education among the people and their ability to read (level of education) understandably improves by fostering a common goal rather than division.

D.O Adeyemo in his study "Local Government and Health Care delivery in Nigeria: A Case Study published in 2005, tries to evaluate the performance of primary health care in Ife-East Local government Area of Nigeria employing empirical, descriptive and survey methods. The author identified the major contradictions in the management of primary health care (PHC) implementation including shortage of qualified personnel and finance, inadequate transportation, inaccessibility to communities, lack of maintenance culture, political instability and high degree of leadership turn-over. For the sustainability of health care service delivery at the grassroots, author recommends increased financial allocation, community mobilization, improved health education, policy consistency, and provision of qualified health workers. He finally concludes that primary health care in Nigeria and especially Ife-East local Government have come a long way and certainly still require more effort so as to achieve the goal of health for all now and beyond.

Nguen Quoc Viet in his own study of deconcentration of rural community government Service intended for the people: "the case of Daknong and Hau-giang Province in Vietnam" published in 2009; the author tries to analyze the rural government community service given in Vietnam in the context of deconcentration process using case study method and decentralization theory. According to the author, the influence of deconcentration changes very much due to the situation of things surrounding the great government establishments and their support system. The author then believes that sustained improvement and supply of basic human needs can influence and quicken the rate of socio-development at every levels of the government. The author concludes that the circumstance of deconcentration of service in Vietnam shows how the services are carried out via the central government to the disadvantage of the rural areas. In this study, Viet argues that rapid development of investment initiatives and physical infrastructure are very important for economic growth but the improvements of local authority capacity in public service delivery are also important for the success of the socio-economic development goals at all levels of governance. Author finally concludes that situation of decentralization in Vietnam still shows that these public goods and services are delivered largely through central institutions due to the weakness of local institution capacity.

M.O. Ojeifo in his study of "Problems of effective Primary Healthcare Delivery in Owan East and Owan West Local Government Areas of Edo State, Nigeria" published 2008, tries to evaluate the performance of primary health care delivery in Owan East and Owan West Local Governments of Edo State, Nigeria. Author identified that primary health centers are the responsibility of the Local government Council that is closest to the people. Nevertheless, how many of these centers are located in a ward depends on population factor and physical size of the ward. He also identified the following factors as obstacles: distance, lack of qualified personnel (inadequacy), equipment shortage, and inadequacies, lack of transportation and good roads, lack of finance and access. Author believes these indeed have increased mortality rate and diseases infection among children and adults in the area. He argues that the lack of infrastructure can only be improved with complementary effort from the federal government. Ojeifo concludes by recommending that the Federal Government should take care of the primary health care in Nigeria in order to keep population alive. Second, is that the Federal Government to and must increase funding to the Local governments to better equip the facilities in place while more personnel can be employed to serve the population. Author finally believes that implementing these recommendations can help public policy makers revamp primary health care in Nigeria.

Andrew G. Onokerhoraye in his study "Access and Utilization of Modern Health Care Facilities in the Petroleum - producing region of Nigeria: A Case Study" published 1999, tries to evaluate the provision of adequate primary health care centers in the state. The paper tries to say that the study shows that the vast proportion of the population of the state has no access to secondary health facilities. The author believes that the success of a deliberate policy of dispersal of primary and secondary health establishments as articulated in the study must be closely related to programs of rural development and settlement upgrading in the southern part of the state. Development planning in Nigeria has focused upon the urban areas at the expense of the rural communities. The author argues that if secondary and to some extent, primary health services are to be attracted and made functional in the rural communities in the area, the availability of essential infrastructure services such as roads and water transport are important. That requires the participation of the people, the private sector, non-governmental organizations, and the federal and state government agencies particularly those responsible for the development of the petroleum producing areas.

The World Bank (2007) study report on "India's Governments and Rural Service Delivery" tries to analyze the issues of performance and functions of the various Indian authorities and their leadership establishments with special programs for supplying the major forms of community needed works and activities. The study focuses only in four key areas which include health, education, drinking water and sanitation, and employment programs covering four selected states (Kerela, Karnataka, West Bengal and Rajasthan) in India.

The study focused mainly on policy question on "What the various levels of Panchayas could do in the delivery of those services within the government structure created by the 1993 Amendment to the constitution of India and relevant state - level legislation". The main findings of the study are the following:

- Consistent with the decentralization to the states, the Constitutional Amendment gives the states the responsibility for creating the enabling environment for local government.
- Legislation defining roles in the service delivery is spread over a large number of legal instruments that often contradict each other, but this is allowed in India's law.
- Centrally sponsored Schemes are highly distortion to the institutional and organizational framework adopted by states in support of decentralization.
- Most states have failed to support devolution of functions with devolution of funds.

- No state has devolved responsibility over functionaries to the local level and together with lacks of funds that handicaps the ability of Panchayas to deliver meaningful services even where legislation assigns to them is the main role.

- Practice on the ground is more centralized than what the legal framework prescribes.

- Service delivery in the rural areas has perverse and systematic problems and outcomes are poor.

Finally, the study concludes that, all services are still largely being provided in the top-down manner through the state civil service, and that services continue to fail the rural poor. Even where services have unequivocally been devolved to the Panchayas, their ability to influence outcomes is limited because of the lack of financial and administrative control.

Zahid Hasnain in his study, "Passing on Responsibility, Explanation and Work Performance: Some Insights from Pakistan", published in 2008, tries to explain the degree of accessibility of local policymakers and the level of competition in local elections, the expenditure patterns of local governments to gauge their sector priorities, and the extent to which local governments are focused on patronage or the provision of targeted benefits to a few as opposed to providing public goods and services. The main findings of the study are threefold. First, the accessibility of policy-makers to citizens in Pakistan is unequivocally greater after devolution, and local government elections are, with some notable exceptions, as competitive as national and provincial elections. Second, Local Government sector priorities are heavily tilted toward the provision of physical infrastructure; specifically, roads, water and sanitation, and rural electrification at the expense of education and health. Third, this sector prioritization is in part a dutiful response to the relatively greater citizen demands for physical infrastructure; in part a reflection of local government electoral structure that gives primacy to village and neighborhood - specific issues, and in part a reaction to provincial initiatives in education and health that have taken the political space away from local governments in the social sectors, thereby encouraging them to focus more toward physical infrastructure.

Inference for Forthcoming Study.

In summary, the above selected set of literature shows that many studies have been done under this particular theme. However, no studies have been done or conducted concerning the newly constituted Owerri and its local government areas, hence this study. In general, the significant commonality here is that looking and considering the Owerri local area issues, the take home here is that although local administration may be similar, but priorities differ. With regards to Owerri case, adequate and affordable healthcare is of utmost priority. However, achieving this is strangled and influenced by Access, Culture and Social networking as indicated by Kleinman (1980) or Social resources (Ikels, 2002).

Above all, the common theme here is that is crucial that the success of a deliberate rural development policy be sustainable whether primary or secondary health facilities or any other developmental project in the rural area be maintained and upgraded with proper functional equipment as well as well trained personnel and community involvement. This will also require adequate leadership that has the capacity and good interest of the people at heart. It will also require good access roads and transportation, and public-private partnership that will make it more attractive for the people's participation. It will also involve more funding from both the state and central governments to make it more sustainable if the goals of the healthcare policies or projects are to be achieved for the proposed area such as Owerri and its locals.

Theoretical/Conceptual Framework for Forthcoming Study

According to the Nigerian constitution, the provision of adequate health care service is a right not a privilege. The neglect, lack of access and inadequate health care service in rural Nigeria remains pathetic and prevalent. This has caused corollary health issues including but not limited to the rise and lack of preventive infections such as malaria, increase in infant mortality rate, increase death in mother and baby with decrease survival rate as earlier noted in this discussion. This research project offers solution and looks at various interventions to help ameliorate the situation as it relates to the obvious gaps and missed opportunities as noted and observed by this study. Hence, the objective of the study includes the description of the factors affecting access, delivery, and utilization of health care delivery in the Owerri locale and its communities.

The Service Delivery Models

The statement of the problem of health care service delivery in Owerri can be examined through the application of Service Delivery Models. United Nations Development Program (UNDP, 1999) defines service delivery as an arranged process by which the government that has the authority over the service uses to deliver it (service) to the people (public). It is this order of establishment for which an organization is put in place that determines the nature of services to be served or supplied to the people. That is to say, that it is the established (institutional) arrangement that is put in place that determines and influences the performance of public service delivery.

The UNDP (1999) highlighted four accepted models of carrying out the function of serving the public based on the delivery arrangements that governments everywhere have adopted. These include:

Direct Service Delivery Model. This is a system where the central government exacts laws and brings out legislation, enforces it by hiring people, invests in them, to carry out the functions or services directly from the central office or through de-concentrated line agencies, assumes full responsibility, and is accountable not only for provisioning but also for delivering services.

Privatization Service Delivery Model. This is a method where the central government (such as the federal government of Nigeria) transfers the delivery of public services to a third party or private companies but retains the ability to supervise, advice and support the process. In this case, it assumes no responsibility except for monitoring the company's compliance to legal codes and standards such as transportation and communication services. The fundamental benefit of this is for the government to lay aside and allow the ability of the market to perform - allocation efficiency. It also helps government to meet up resource gaps in service delivery to the people.

Alternative Service Delivery Model. In the arena of public administration, the "Alternative Service Delivery Model" is a relatively recent phenomenon. This model brings together the government and private sector under various contractual arrangements. However, the ultimate ownership is generally vested within the government, which retains the power to provide public services, whereas the private parties make the actual delivery.

Decentralization Service Delivery Model. Decentralization or simply decentralization service delivery is a simple system or method of transferring works or functions to the local or rural government bodies. It is the method with the understanding that lower level of administration is closer to the people and will therefore do the job better, hence the most popular model in most countries.

The Meaning of Decentralization

Decentralization means transfer of power, authority, responsibilities, and functions from the central government to local or sub national units of the government. It has been defined by various scholars as transference of authority from a higher level of government to a lower one, delegation of decision making, placement of authority with responsibility allowing greatest number of actions to be taken where most of the people reside, removal of functions from the center to the periphery, a mode of operations involving wider participation of people in the whole range of decision making beginning from plan formulation to implementation (Akramove, 2008; Rahman & Khan, 1996). There are three essential characteristics of decentralization:

- The greatest number of decisions should be made in the field; officers must be selected and trained as to develop the capacity to resolve the problem on the spot.

- A decentralized administration must be developed as far as possible with the active participation of the people themselves. Their cooperation and compliance are essential and the services of the state and the local agencies supplementing and stimulating but not duplicating their staff or equipment should be utilized.

- Coordination of the work of the various agencies in the field should be done in the field itself because; central coordination means delays, jealousies, and jurisdictional disputes (Rahman, et al, 1997).

Forms of Decentralization

Decentralization is a comprehensive concept that takes many forms. Scot (2002) has identified three major forms, namely de-concentration, delegation and devolution, which are discussed below.

Deconcentration. Deconcentration indicates the redistribution of administrative powers and responsibilities only within the central government. A process that involves the transfer of functions within the central government hierarchy through the shifting of the workload from central ministries to field offices, the creation of field agencies, or the shifting of the responsibility to local administrative units that are part of central government structure.

Delegation. Delegation refers to transfer of powers or functions to organizations that are not under the direct control of central government ministries. It implies the transfer or creation of broad authority to play and implement decisions concerning specific activities within specific spatial boundaries to an organization that is technically and administratively capable of carrying them out without direct supervision by a higher administrative unit.

Devolution. Devolution is the preferred form of decentralization and it refers to transfer of full power and responsibility for delivery of public goods and services to local governments, who have legislative, revenue-raising, and decision-making powers. Rahaman et al. (1997) clarified the process of devolution by identifying five fundamental characteristics:

- Powers are transferred to autonomous local units governed independently without the direct control of the center.
- The local governments are given legal powers to exercise authority over a recognized geographical area.
- The local units have corporate status and power to secure resources to perform their functions.
- Devolution implies the need to develop local governments and institutions.
- It is a process of reciprocal, mutually beneficial, and coordinated relationships between central and local governments.

It should be pointed out that there are additional forms of decentralization that exist in theory. The review of the literature for this study suggests that there is no tangible evidence to indicate successful or effective policy outcomes garnered from the implementation of these alternate models.

Dimensions of Decentralization

Decentralization can be examined in terms of several dimensions. According to Akramov (2008) and Manor (1997), there are three dimensions of decentralization, namely political, administrative (institutional) and fiscal decentralization.

Political Decentralization

Political decentralization is the transfer of authority to a sub - national body. Political decentralization aims to give citizens or their elected representatives more power in public decision making. It is often associated with pluralistic and representative government, but it can also support democratization by giving citizens, or their representatives, more influence in the formulation and implementation of policies. Political decentralization assumes that decisions made with greater participation will be better informed and more relevant to diverse interest in society than those made only by national political authorities. The concept implies that the selection of representations from local electoral jurisdictions allows entireness to know better their political representatives and allows elected officials to know better the needs and desires of their constituents. Political decentralization often requires constitutional or statutory reforms, the development of pluralistic political parties, the strengthening of legislatures, creations of local political units, and the encouragement of effective public interest groups.

Administrative Decentralization

Administrative decentralization implies the transfer of responsibility for planning, management, and the raising and allocation of resources from the central government and its agencies to field units of government agencies, subordinate units of levels of government, semi-autonomous public authorities or corporations, area wide, regional, or functional authorities, or non-governmental private or voluntary organizations.

Fiscal Decentralization

Fiscal decentralization implies the transfer of financial responsibility in as far as the generating of revenue as well as authority to make expenditure decisions from the central government to the lower levels of government. This is a core component of decentralization, as the discharge of devolved functions by the local governments requires matching financial resources from the central government. It must, however, be stressed that all the dimensions are cardinal in ensuring that the goals of decentralization are achieved and that all three operate in an interdependent fashion albeit the fiscal aspect is critical (Pradeep, 2011).

Reasons for Providing Decentralized Services

There are perceived advantages and disadvantages of decentralization on service delivery. If well-designed and implemented, it is argued that decentralization could have advantages on service delivery including:

- Facilitating good governance by empowering the local population and allowing them to participate in matters affecting their lives. This allows the local people to be a watchdog on the system and ensure that the public officials deliver quality goods and services (World Bank, 2000).

- Improving service delivery. It is argued that the lower levels of government can deliver services such as water, education, sanitation, healthcare, etc more effectively. Also, at the lower levels of government, politicians and civil servants are more aware of the needs of their community making them more responsive in providing such services. Preferences of local populations are better be known at lower levels of government (Predeep, 2011).

- The productive efficiency argument. This refers to the contention that local governments can produce the same goods and services at lower costs than central governments. Because sub-national governments are closer to the population, cost of producing goods and services will be minimal.

- The usual 'middle-men syndrome' and bureaucracy involving contract procedures would be reduced

- Improving the efficiency of central governments. Decentralization allows central governments to concentrate on national and international issues. The central government can concentrate on macroeconomic policies for the entire economy rather than being pre-occupied with delivering services to all the communities.

- Decentralization may make it less difficult for government to recover the costs of public services. That is, services would be more demand responsive hence increasing the households' willingness to pay for services. In other words, households and their families are perceived to be more willing to pay for and maintain services that match their demand.

- Fostering competition may result in better public goods at lower prices. "Competition allows a variety of bundles of local public goods to be produced and individuals can reveal their preferences for those goods by exercising some form of 'exit' option at the extreme, moving to those jurisdictions that satisfy their tastes" (Azfar, 2005).

- Decentralized units may need less professionalization and can engage manpower from civil society thus administration costs will be lower and procedures simpler.

Disadvantages of Decentralization

Unless it is thoughtfully designed and effectively implemented, decentralization may not be a panacea for all the service delivery illnesses in the developing world. It is argued that decentralization could have disadvantages on service delivery including:

- Lack of capacity at sub-national levels of government in exercising responsibility for public services. In Uganda and Tanzania, the lower tiers of government lacked the ability to manage public finances and maintain proper accounting procedures. Consequently, lower levels of government received less money than before decentralization (Ahmad et al, 2005).

- Decentralization may result in misaligned responsibilities either due to incomplete process or for political reasons. For example, in Nigeria, under the Universal Basic Education (UBE) program, the Federal Government releases money to State Primary School Boards but cannot hire, fire, replace or evaluate teachers (Ahmad et al, 2005).

- Decentralization has led to corruption of the lower levels of government partly due to weaker accountability and transparency issues.

- There are problems tangentially related to decentralization. For example, the "soft-judges constraint confronting sub-national governments may lead to over borrowing". The social impact of the Argentina crises at the end of 2001 resulted in the deterioration of service quality: poverty rates jumped 40 percent, medical supplies were in short supply in almost all the public hospitals and there were many school closings during the year (World Bank, 2003).

The Purpose of Decentralization Service

It is believed that decentralization is based on subsidiary principles of governance; a rule where provision, production and delivery of services are to be devolved to the lowest governmental tier, local or rural bodies who subject to economies of scale and capacity. By virtue of being closest to the citizens, local bodies are better positioned to match supply of a given service to citizens' demands, thereby transforming citizens from service recipient to client, and ensuring citizens greater accountability for service quality.

Multi-Level Governance Model

According to Stubbs (2005), this is a system of government model that promotes neo-pluralism, meaning that it recognizes the presence and participation of different networks and political communities in the decision-making process, besides the interest of old groups and problems are solved after reaching a compromise through the mixture (aggregation) of the various divergent interests. It has also been described as a multi-tiered governance, polycentric governance and multi-perspective governance.

It signifies the totality of relations between public and private sector actors, situated at different territorial levels in the governance process. Marks (1993) originally defended the model of MLG as a system of continuous negotiation among nested governments at several territorial tiers which are supranational, national, regional and local governments are enmeshed in territorially overarching policy networks. Jachtenfuchs (1995) extended this institutional definition to encompass "the relationships between governance processes and different government levels". Bache and Flinders (2004) admit that currently there is no single widely embraced definition of the model of MLG; however they identify four common strands in the research carried out under its aegis. These are:

- The tendency over time to increasing participation of non-state actors such as Non-governmental Organization (NGOs), corporations and unions in governance functions.
- The proliferation of overlapping decision-making networks engaged in such functions.
- The change in the role of the state from command and control to steering, coordination and networking.
- The challenges MLG confronts in assigning responsibility and in exercising democratic accountability in governance.

The objective of governance consists of the involvement of all the actors, through different forms of partnership, regardless of the level at which they are situated (community institutions, national governments, local and regional authorities or civil society). A specific feature of the MLG system is the fact that the decision-making process is based on negotiations between the main actors, to arrive at a consensus and non-majority vote.

Dimensions of Multi-Level Governance

The MLG model can be looked at in terms of several dimensions. Patrick and et al (2005) have distinguished two major dimensions, namely horizontal dimension and vertical dimension.

The horizontal dimension refers to the opening up of the political space to non-state actors, meaning that the State now has to interact with non-state actors (civil society and business community) in the governance process. In other words, government has to 'produce' governance by taking into account the desiderata of a multiplicity of stakeholders. It also has to provide room and resources to these stakeholders for the realization of public policy goals.

The vertical dimension refers to both the upward and downward decision-making Processes. The upward process is one in which national decision-making process is concerned with the supranational decision-making process. The downward process is a method of using decentralization, particularly the devolution of power to pass on their obligation in the process of organizing the issues. As such, MLG involves the existence of multiple political decision-making centers at different levels (sub-national, national, supranational, international) as connected among themselves at different political levels. Thus, by realizing that political interdependence means that the political process at one level influences the political processes or outcomes at other levels and vice versa.

Types of Multi-Level Governance

MLG model also can be looked at in terms of several types. Hooghe and Marks (2003) subdivided the MLG model into two types, which they labeled Type I and Type II. Type I MLG has several distinctive characteristics. The number of levels of governance is limited to no more than five, including the international, regional supranational, national, constituent sub-national, and local. These are generally defined in territorial rather than functional terms. Each of these levels has general-purpose jurisdictions that "amalgamates multiple functions", including a range of policy responsibilities, and in many cases, a court system and representative institutions.

The jurisdictions are nonintersecting in membership, and there is only one relevant jurisdiction at each territorial scale. They note that although the jurisdictions tend to be stable, there is flexibility in the allocation of policy competences within them.

Although the inspiration for these Type I systems of MLG is federalism, they are not limited to this governance form, or even to its identification with the nation-state.

Type II MLG is defined primarily in functional terms. It consists of special-purpose jurisdictions or policy structures that are highly fragmented and numerous. The authors also believe that they tend to be ephemeral, flexible and variable in nature.

Critique of Multi-Level Governance

The MLG model has been subjected to critical analysis and debate during the past decade. The following perspectives serve as a summary of noteworthy opinions regarding the efficacy and viability of the model.

The MLG model does have the merit of emphasizing the changing influence on decision-making of different actors in different policy sectors and at different levels of governance. However, it tends to exaggerate the importance of sub-national actors and to neglect the implementation and outcome stage of policy-making, in which national governments have a particularly important role, and in which the MLG pattern is most prevalent. Bache (1998), expressed that national governments continue to play a central "gate-keeping" role at all stages of policy-making and in all policy sectors, whereas actors from the supranational and sub-national levels are merely participants, not actual decision-makers, in this process.

The MLG model is prone to exaggerate the hierarchical and legal nature of intergovernmental relationships prior to the emergence of genuine MLG. In addition, they are inclined to overemphasize what they call the "post-constitutional" and "extra-constitutional" nature of MLG. They see MLG, somewhat artificially, as "a model of governance that largely defies, or ignores, structure", disregards or downplays institutions, and concentrates almost entirely on processes and outcomes. In that sense, it lacks a clear conceptual focus (Peters and Pierre, 2004).

The MLG model tends to give priority to the objective of problem-solving capacity rather than democratic input and accountability. Peters and Pierre (2004) describe this as a "Faustian bargain" in which "the core values of democratic government are traded for accommodation, consensus, and efficiency in governance," in which informal patterns of shared decision-making may disguise "a strategy for political interests to escape or bypass regulations intended to limit their freedom of action. The MLG model is often attacked for being too descriptive. It is seen as unable to explain or predict governance policy outcomes.

The Purpose of the Multi-Level Governance Model

In spite of critical viewpoints, the MLG model suggests that there is a rather wide array of specific determinants that influence consumer decisions to seek health care services in Owerri. Culture, economics, access to health care, perception, knowledge, belief in efficacy, tradition, age , gender roles, and social roles are among the factors that impact both steps in the decision-making process: The decision to seek health care services; and, the choice regarding which specific form of health care to seek for preventive care or for the treatment of a current illness.

The Medical Choice-Making Model.

To understand behavioral and perceptional factors that influence how healthcare services are accessed by Owerri residents and provided to them by Owerri healthcare providers, this study has taken into consideration the following theoretical construct and applied model of medical choice-making model.

- Young (1981) proposed a choice-making model which is based on his Ethnographic studies of health services utilization in Mexico (Figure 1). This model incorporates four components that are most essential to the individual's health service choice as related to the Owerri population:

- Perceptions of gravity of illness. This category includes both the individual's perception and their social network's consideration of illness severity. Gravity is based on the assumption that the culture classifies illnesses by level of severity;

- The knowledge of a cultural, traditional, or home treatment or remedy. If a person knows of a Home (or traditional) remedy that is efficacious, they will be likely to utilize that home treatment before utilizing a professional health care system. Home remedy knowledge is based on lay referral;

- The faith in remedy for illness. This component incorporates the individual's belief of efficacy of treatment for the present illness. An individual will not utilize the treatment if they do not believe the treatment is effective;

- The accessibility of treatment. Accessibility incorporates the individual's evaluation of the cost of health services and the availability of those services - which when lacking as in Owerri particularly long term, may convince people to try and use the home or traditional remedy they know or deem possible which may not be appropriate. According to Young, access may be the most important influence on health care utilization (Wolinsky, 1988b).

Recognizing Choice: Model Building

According to the choice-making medical model and literature review in considering the Owerri healthcare issues, three components of threats to seek health care emerged. The described choice-making model and literature review contain threads of commonality via three factors that influence the process of health care seeking in Owerri:

- Health care access;
- Culture; and
- Social networks.

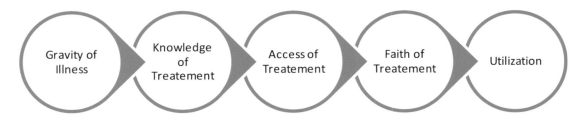

Figure 1. Young's Choice Making Model.

Access describes the ability to utilize services and incorporates economics, geographic location, abundance of health services, and physical and social resources. If health services are not accessible, it is likely that there will be unmet needs for health care service for the people (as in Owerri). Next, culture is a complex term referring to values, practices, meanings, and beliefs that are transmitted from one person to another through the process of enculturation. Culture, often considered a barrier to health services, can influence knowledge and beliefs of illness as well as the course of treatment for illness. Last in interacting with culture, is social networks that can also cue an individual to utilize or abstain from health services and can function in identification of illness and illness response. While other elements certainly affect health care utilization, exploring these three concepts is central to understanding determinants of health care utilization in Owerri.

First, the economic costs of health care seeking include not only payment for treatment, but also lost productive time, and the expense of transportation (especially rural Owerri). Unless provided with a subsidized health care plan, persons of lower socioeconomic status can have difficulty affording the costs associated with utilization of health care, making utilization less likely (Taylor, 2003). Similarly, due to the expense of transportation and time needed to access medical care, especially as health care services become more geographically scarce or distant (as in Owerri), inaccessibility may increase (Young & Young-Garro, 1982).

Accessibility of health care is further influenced by physical and social resources. For instance, in individuals who have suffered debilitating injuries, geographic location can become an impediment to the use of health care services (LaVela, Smith, Weaver, & Miskevics, 2004). Moreover, beyond physical limitations, social resources are also integral to health care services utilization. Social resources include family economic capital, social support, and group knowledge of illnesses and illness treatments. For example, among Taiwanese, Kleinman (1980) found that if an individual's family has knowledge of an effective home remedy the person will often attempt that treatment before utilizing professional health care services. In Kleinman's study, families in Taiwan provided social resources, specifically knowledge, of which a lone ill person may not have been aware, hence, the social support. Thus, the knowledge and social support available to an individual can affect accessibility of specific health care services delivery.

Second, culture shapes not only illness treatment, but also illness recognition, perception of illness severity, and confidence in the efficacy of specific treatments for specific illnesses. For example, in many cultures, dementia in elderly is viewed as a normal process of aging; thus it does not necessitate medical treatment. However, in the United States, dementia is considered an illness requiring professional medical care (Ikels, 2002). As such, variance in health care utilization can result due to cultural knowledge and understandings of illness. Likewise, categories and perceptions of illness are often cultural. Conceptual-incompatibility is a hypothesis frequently used to explain why members of another culture refuse to utilize health care services. A person with conceptual-incompatibility would be unlikely to utilize available health care because the treatment conflicts with their culturally rooted knowledge of illness (Young & Young-Garro, 1982). For example, if a person staunchly believes they are infected with influenza yet are told by a healer that they are actually infected with malaria; the person may not have faith in the treatment prescribed. If a person lacks confidence in the ability for a healer to treat their illness, they may be unlikely to visit this healer for further treatment. As such, belief in the efficacy of treatment, influenced by cultural categories of illness, can shape adherence to prescribed treatment and ultimately the use of health care services.

Beyond faith in efficacy and inadequate education, cultures can have differing notions of the self which may influence health services utilization. For instance, in the United States as well as many other western nations, there are two main conceptions of self, one that is autonomous and one that is heteronymous (Gaines, 1992). If an individual is a member of a culture that considers the self as heteronymous, they are likely to have their course of treatment determined by people within their social network (Kleinman, 1980; Ikels, 2002). Conversely, if a culture considers the individual as autonomous, the decisions for treatment are more likely to be made by the individual. In those cultures that consider the self as heteronymous, an ill individual's treatment may be delayed as persons within their social network discuss treatment options (Janzen, 1978).Yet, even in cultures that stress autonomy, the individual may consult social networks for illness advice. Social networks can provide an impetus for health care utilization but may also press an individual to abstain from accessing health services.

Suchman's concept of parochial and cosmopolitan networks is useful here in considering the effects of social networks. According to Suchman, parochial networks are those that are traditional, close in affiliation, and reluctant to accept new information (Wolinsky, 1988b). Because of their emphasis on tradition, these networks are theoretically likely to utilize home based treatments before scientific based health care such as professional biomedicine. However, persons belonging to cosmopolitan networks are more progressive, willing to accept new information, and more likely to have a scientific approach to illness. As a result, cosmopolitan network members would be more likely to use biomedical health care. Therefore, social networks affect illness knowledge and patterns of health care utilization. As an individual experiences illness, he or she will often consult their network in an effort to identify the illness and the best course of treatment or prevention (Cockerham, 1982).

Finally, other than diseases for which a person believes himself or herself to be at risk, the model tends to disregard utilization of health care services just for maintaining a healthy lifestyle. As a result, people may access health care services simply to maintain their health, not because they perceive themselves as being susceptible to a specific disease (as the case may be).

Understanding Healthcare Service Delivery and the Cultural Influence of Its Application in Owerri

To drive the concept home for the people of Owerri, I introduce the concept of "The Old Automobile Syndrome" (researcher's experience). This concept has five elements involved. Like the automobile (the automobile or car is very familiar to the people of Owerri both old and young), the human body is made of different parts and organs that resemble the automobile make up that need regular tune ups, repairs (self), and maintenance like the old automobile.

So, the human parts need similar routine checks, repairs, maintenance and nourishment to have the energy to function and work normally, else they will detach and malfunction – sickness (like a faulty car). Thus, understanding that just as a sick car needs a mechanic for attention, the sick needs a qualified health care professionals (doctors, nurses, etc.) to do same in a similar and following ways:

- Needs a professional attention to evaluate the sick condition;
- Diagnose and evaluate the condition;

- Needs a professional treatment and attention;

- Needs the proper management of the outcome of the evaluation (which includes the discussion on choice and treatment options);

- The treatment option depends on the general family consensus, payment capability, leadership and relationship with the social network (which could be cultural or traditional, autonomous, heterogeneous, parochial or cosmopolitan.

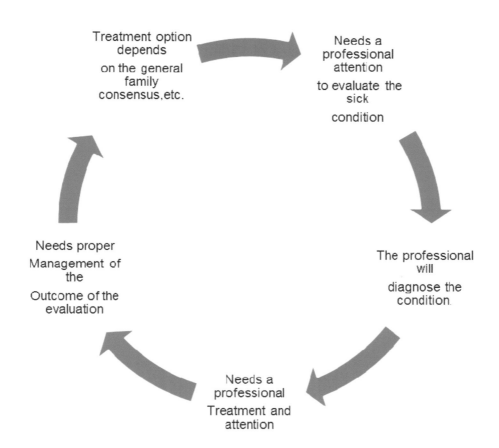

Figure 2. Care services delivery and cultural influence of application in Owerri.

Adapted and Modified from the Old Automobile Model

As a result, receiving health care service, medical service or utilization is delayed in most cases or too late when accepted which may lead to negative outcome or untoward effect. Because the population is mainly rural and to an extent compounded by poor roads and lack of available transportation, the inadequacy of healthcare staff, professionals and facilities, the result could be deadly and with a resounding disappointment (as noted in this paper that shows the morbidity and population growth rates). Therefore, proper education and the importance of health care services delivery and the utilization of available services, resources and facilities become paramount within Owerri, around the state and Nigeria as a whole. For example, recently the First Lady of Nigeria (Mrs. Jonathan who was transferred to Germany for medical treatment) was misdiagnosed by the presidential physicians as mystery around ailment grows (City Flames, September 7, 2012). Thus, there are significant unmet needs for health care as a whole. According to Einthoven and Vorhause (1997), the knowledge, judgment, and skill of the physician are the single most important determinants of the quality of health care. Completion of a residency and achievement of licensure do not ensure that a physician has these qualities. Ideally, a high quality health care organization attracts the loyalty, commitment, and responsible participation of good knowledgeable physicians that can make well-informed decisions about their clients and consumers in their ability to satisfying their needs. The case of the Current Nigeria's First Lady is a good testimony of the case in point.

With a better understanding of why people use or do not use these services, health care organizations can seek to improve the quality of health in Owerri and Imo State as noted earlier. Therefore, the failure to utilize health care services was a consequence of perceived needs, perceived threats, illness knowledge, autonomous health care choices, and faith in treatment as highlighted in the discussion. As such, the unmet need for health care is growing especially in the face of growing Owerri and Nigeria population, a startling threat to quality of life. Identifying the factors that prevent and spur the use of health care services in Owerri including the use of alternative medicines (for instance Chiropractor, acupuncture, herbal remedies and other healers) not normally offered by biomedical practitioners will ultimately help health care organizations create programs for improving health services and increasing their utilization. As a result, health care organizations in Owerri and around the State including the government must discern the factors influencing health care utilization. Identifying who will use which services and when these services will be used can help organizations target consumers for medical contact.

Importantly, according to the population projection, Owerri is becoming more diverse with increasing cultural heterogeneity as well (researcher's experience). Hence, healthcare delivery and utilization is likely to shift as well. Addressing the needs of this shifting and diverse population requires an understanding of the culturally linked health care utilization determinants as well. In addition, this knowledge can also help health care organizations and their leaders identify new customers, spot concerns of consumers who are rejecting health services, and ultimately increase customer satisfaction. Also understanding why people utilize alternative or conventional medicines is central to increasing health care delivery, utility and efficacy in Owerri (and around the state) due to culture, cost and education as already discussed or referenced to address the issues.

Similarly, another population trend is in aging. Life expectancy in nearly every nation has increased. In 2000, the World Health Organization noted that global life expectancy was 65.5 years, nearly six years longer than in 1980 (Bonita & Mathers, 2003). Moreover, by 2050, there will be approximately two billion people over the age of 60, and the global median age will have increased from 28 in 2007 to 38 (United Nations Department of Economic and Social Affairs, 2007). Elderly tend to utilize health care resources more often than people under the age of 65. As such, the shift in demographics should be an indicator that utilization of health services is likely to increase. However, despite increased likelihood of use, there are many determinants which can create unmet needs for health services. For example, physical disability has been shown to be a significant predictor of health care utilization among the elderly. Elderly who are disabled are less likely to access care than are physically healthy older adults (Linden, Horgas, Gilberg, & Steinhagen-Thiessen, 1997). Although seemingly self explanatory, as global population continues to age, health care organizations must recognize the determinants and impediments to health care utilization including that of Owerri, Imo State and Nigeria as a whole.

The Infrastructural Planning and Development Model

Meaning of Infrastructure

Infrastructural facilities refer to those basic services without which primary, secondary, and tertiary productive activities cannot function. In its wider application, infrastructural activities embrace all public services from law and order through to education and public health to transportation, communication, and water supply. The infrastructural approach to rural or local development is one method commonly used by most Third World countries. Abumere (2002) defined rural infrastructure to include the system of physical, human, and institutional forms of capital which enables rural residents to better perform their production, processing, and distribution activities, as well as help to improve the overall quality of life. Some of these infrastructures are roads, communication network, irrigation, storage facilities, research and extension institutions, schools, and universities that train and turn out a variety of skilled and agricultural workers.

Nigeria, as in other developing countries, is linked to the antecedents of development dating to the colonial era as noted below. According to Onimode (1988) given Nigeria's colonial and neo-colonial historical experiences which culminated in the rural - urban inequality in the distribution of socio-economic facilities, the majority of rural populace are trapped and sub-merged in a sub-human culture of silence, misery, and isolation. Unreliable access feeder roads, no light or epileptic power supply, no basic health facility, no decent housing, no major educational institution, no recreational facilities among others, characterize many parts of rural Nigeria (Olayiwola & Adeleye, 2005). In other words, infrastructural facilities are the elements in the package of basic needs that a community (like a rural area such as Owerri locales) would like to procure for better living.

The Purpose of Infrastructural Planning and Development Model

According to Oguzor (2011), in any nation, growth and development, whether in urban or rural (local) setting, are consequent on the availability of the infrastructure that provide the essential utilities and services necessary for improved standard of living. There is a need for infrastructural development in urban and local or rural areas, especially with the latter being grossly neglected until more recently as exemplified by literature (Okali, Okpara, & Olowoye, 2001). The authors believe that in the country of Nigeria infrastructural facilities and services that form the bedrock foundation of rural planning, development and progress depends on the provision and availability of those amenities that induces population, agglomeration, and growth, the basic footing on which development activities stand as well as the principal ingredients for the development process are poorly developed.

The Consequences of Lack of Infrastructural Planning and Development

As noted above, the authors believe that the lack of these amenities to meet the basic needs of the suburbia is the fundamental cause of the rural-urban migration. Hence, improving and providing the necessities of life in the suburbs will help alleviate the dichotomy of both service and development. This phenomenal process is crucial in the rural area improvement, and an understandable knowledge of the issue becomes essential for rural development. As a result, this research project pays attention to the provision and affordability of quality healthcare to the Owerri local population as one of the major factors missing and lacking in the process.

The inadequate provision of such services as electricity supply, pipe-borne water supply, health care services, and more readily available modes of transport and communication in rural areas will militate against prospects for better living standards and prospects for employment and other forms of economic activities becomes the lighting rod of the subject matter. Thus, the great importance the issue of rural or local infrastructure has assumed in recent times is indicative of the failure of past efforts. An awareness of their importance is a key to rural or local development of health improvement.

Theory of Organizational Change:

Introduction

According to Cummings, et al (2005), organizational change or transformation can be defined as activities directed at changing the basic characteristics of the organization. It focuses on change triggered by the societal dynamics change. It also involves implementing some new ways or plans to improve the relationship between the local executives and the people as a whole that requires expert intervention. This research project focuses on the special case of change or transformation triggered by the leadership dynamics change. Implementing some of the new ways in which to improve the relationships between the local leadership executives and the people (public) as a whole becomes important. The change theory here explores and highlights the need for change in order to make progress and benefit the people of Owerri. Hence, the implementation of the new change becomes necessary taking into account those steps needed to effect the change. Therefore, as a team the people have to implement an organizational transformation that will help interpret and implement the findings of what is happening at the organizational level.

The Lewin's Theory of Change

The change theory applied in this project is the Lewin's theory of change. According to Cummings & Worley (2005), Lewin conceived of change as modification of those forces keeping a system's behavior stable. Specifically, a particular set of behaviors at any moment in time is the result of two groups of forces: those pushing for change (like the people of Owerri) and those striving to maintain the status quo (the state and Nigerian Governments) thus, maintaining the equilibrium. To change the state of equilibrium, one can increase those forces pushing for change, decrease those forces maintaining the current state of things, or apply some combination of both. This level can be increased either by changing the group norms to support higher levels of performance or by increasing pressures on the management and administrative leadership to produce at higher levels. According to the authors, Lewin suggested that modifying those forces maintaining the status quo produces less tension on the process and resistance than increasing forces for the change and consequently is a more effective change strategy.

The authors state that Lewin's theory of planned change process consists of three steps as follows:

- **Unfreezing.** This involves change for people to let go the old way of doing business or things by finding a way to change. By overcoming the opposing activities, plans, or driving forces that could hinder moving beyond the current situation of things or the status quo to achieve change. This means finding a new driving level of forces to shift the bar to a new line of change at a new level of equilibrium that becomes the change by definition or itself.

- **Moving.** This process involves thought, feeling, behavior, action, attitude, and ideas that move above the old level of things or situation to cause change.

- **Refreezing.** This process opens up a new avenue making it possible to move on to establish a new strategic equilibrium level that becomes the new change and habit or routine standard.

- **Application.** It is important to note that implementing the planned change needs evaluation and proper analysis. This is achieved by applying the SWOT analysis.

According to Cummings & Worley (2005), leadership is defined as a process of influence exercised when institutional, political, psychological, and other resources are used to arouse, engage, and satisfy the motives of followers. It can also be seen as the art of mobilizing the interest, energy and commitment of all people at all levels of an organization. Therefore, an effective leader knows that the ultimate task of leadership is to create energies and human vision for the follower or people in the organization or relationship that are lacking in the case of Owerri experience. By so doing, the issue of leadership and achieving extra ordinary things, motivating and influencing the people is lacking in the Owerri experience. As a result, there is no clear vision from the local leaders to set visionary direction for the people they serve or even to inspire them for a better future. Hence, they are only interested in their personal gains and giving rise to corruption.

In addition, the local leaders also lack the emotional support and connection with the people they serve. Maybe they need to walk in the shoes of the people to be able to comprehend the sentiments of the people in order to understand their plight and favorably communicate with and connect to them.

Above all, the lack of empathy can obviously instill bad blood between the two parties which can choke the relationship even further. The bad relationship undoubtedly can obscure and stiffen communication between leadership and the followers (people) which makes matters even worst between the two. As a resolution, it is also important for leadership to own up to their mistakes so that the people or followers can find closure to the issues of wrong doing and move on with their lives. This can be meaningfully important as to rebuild credibility, confidence, and trust within and among the involved parties.

Reason for Change

The following are some of the reasons that can initiate and cause change including but not limited to:

- Change can be triggered by societal, environmental and internal disruption.

- By public discontinuities such as change in leadership, political landscape, economic change, and technological conditions that shift the basis for competition within the organization or the community such as Owerri.

- Government policy shift change: Changes in program due to government policy that requires different business strategies and methods of implementation or doing business (as in Owerri health care production).

- Internal politics and political change, leadership and organizational change, societal dynamics: changes in size, executive turnover and rough or tough economic times, etc. (as affecting Owerri and the state of Imo).

The Solution for Change

These will include the following:

- Earning the people's interest, trust, support, cooperation and understanding.
- Long-term planning to modify programs, procedures, policies and some other necessary methods within the Systems.
- Soliciting rapid implementation of programs and policies of change needed by the people to ensure immediate competitive survival - this is the key for the whole organizational overhaul, hence believing that the move made will make a big difference.
- Ensuring measurable increase in general organizational performance within the system with an anticipatory goal of 100%.
- Defining organizational goals and objectives.
- Mentoring and good membership support with respect, building bonds by trying to make amends through understanding, accommodating, accepting and apologizing to followers or the people by the leadership when there is mistake.
- It may also be helpful and reasonable for leadership to empower the people to take action to defend their right as needed when necessary through the participatory leadership role.

The Benefits of Change

The benefits of the change include but not limited to:

Achieving one voice and working together as a team.

- Leads to organizational realignment between the people and the organizational leadership.
- Leads to power recognition with improved efficiency.
- Leads to improved organizational learning process and cooperation through teamwork.

- Leads to confidence development, better planning, and increases outcome and organizational satisfaction.

- It improves communication and trust between leadership and the public.

- Builds team support system, sustains support and strength needed for staying the change course.

Problems Associated with Change

Some of the problems associated with this kind of decision making process Include:

- Lack of agreement on what to do or how to implement the program if at all.

- Causes lack of communication, respect, cooperation, poor service that can affect bottom line and thereby lead to more layoffs disruptions such as disobedience, mistrust, political unrest, layoffs, etc.

- It can also cause change in healthcare that can affect patient care as well.

- It can cause and lead to lack of commitment, mistrust, low productivity, low staff morale, and quitting of the boss instead of the job, which are all very crucial for organizational survival.

Summary

The main lesson here is that organizational leaders should always listen to the people, communicate with them, hear what they are saying and try to be proactive. In essence, whatever constraints that may exist, they are never as serious as the threat to a leader's effectiveness from followers who do not feel a sense of connection and as a result do not follow. Hopefully, any kind of resolution will help restore trust, confidence, respect, commitment, credibility and good working relationship between the two parties as a whole for better outcomes.

SWOT Analysis and Application

This paper briefly talks about the SWOT analysis as noted here. It is primarily used and applied to the business world for analysis. Its application and importance can assist organizations evaluate internal and external threats to success and overall progress. It shows how strategic plans can be made based on the issues identified during the analysis. It then goes on to define the process and show how organizations and individuals alike can apply this tool for both success and survival. In addition, it looks at the problems, solution, the benefits, the learning application, and finally the conclusion as it relates to organizational management and control.

The Process of SWOT Analysis

The risk facing and affecting organizations and their operations today, whether strategic, financial, or operational, can be either external or internal factors or both. Regardless of which of these problems do exist, SWOT analysis will apply and will have similar impacts. Therefore, performing SWOT analysis is the foundation for identifying manageable organizational issues early enough before disaster strikes. Hence, is a method organizations (big and small) can employ and use to identify and manage both external and internal problems. As a result, its relative importance generates this discussion. According to Robertson (2003), SWOT analysis is a method for examining the strength (S), the weakness (W), opportunities (O), and threats (T) facing an organization in the market place or in any other particular situation that needs analysis or evaluation option.

Therefore, it gives the organization an insight of its position in a particular situation in the market place or industry compared with its competitors. Thus, it guides the organization in the following ways: S= strength: This occurs when the organization considers its strong points or core competencies from its own standpoint. It also includes the opinions of the customers' point of view and why they do business with the company; W = weakness. Although this is difficult to think of or talk about, it is also important to equally discuss. It evaluates the company's weakness not only from their own perspective but also that of their customers as well so that things can improve and done better. O = opportunities: This looks at areas that can offer the company room for growth. It can come from technology and market changes, government policies relating to the industry, changes in demography or general life style changes, etc. These conditions can be explored, exploited and taken advantage of whether locally, nationally or internationally to better position the organization. Finally, T = threats. Traditionally, we do not think about it but we face threats in our business every day. Many times they are out of the organization's reach and control such as the current downturn of the economy, shift in demography, lifestyle changes or perhaps a new mega corporation nearby.

In addition, the analysis includes identifying other obstacles that people such as Owerri and its people face or have but may not know it. For example, is there anything the people can offer or have that can be easily removed or transferred out? Who can do this in the area? What competitions do exist in the area? The SWOT analysis tries to evaluate all these circumstances surrounding the people or organization so that strategic plans can be made and put in place to address the identified issues. Summarize it to say that it is a solution to every problem regardless whether business or people related.

Benefits of SWOT Analysis

Some of the benefits of SWOT analysis here becomes eminent and include the following:

- It helps in taking a close look at things to identify problem areas within the organization ahead of time so that changes could be made for improvement.
- It can help focus leadership on how to improve organizational performance;
- It helps in planning and formulating goals, set priorities, clarify roles and address readiness for change.
- It can also help to identify alternatives and opportunities for organizational growth and survival.

Problems Associated with SWOT Analysis

Some of the risks or problems noted include but not limited to:

- Financial impact that can be significant in terms of planning and implementing new goals and objectives identified.
- It is also difficult identifying organizational weaknesses and threats while opportunities may be lacking or lagging.
- Sometimes, implementing strategies to address identified issues and constraints can be hindered by a centralized government due to power control as in the case of the Owerri experience.

Solutions Associated with SWOT Analysis

The solution here is to solve the above listed problems involving risk taking. To do this means to understand how the people and their organizations can use SWOT analysis to achieve sustainable solutions, hence they should use the benefits of analysis in the following ways in approaching these problems:

- The organization should use its strength to explore and exploit opportunities available to it in anything it is doing to its own advantage.
- It should also use its strength to defeat and defuse threats in order to stay and remain on course.

- The organization should also try to minimize its weakness by taking advantage of available opportunities by identifying other potential alternatives and possibilities for growth better, and expansion thereby creating and bringing new possibilities for the people and to the market place. Thus, generating new revenue string for growth and more opportunities from the new wealth and leverage its overall position.

Learning Application of SWOT Analysis

The lesson here is that the SWOT analysis is flexible and open for anybody and anyone to use whether personal or organizational in nature. However, the main issue is that organizations need it and should use it more to develop strategic plans for dealing with organizational threats that tend to prevent sustained growth and progress for the people and in the market place as well.

The Summary of SWOT Analysis

In summary, it is important to note that organizational knowledge, ideas are changing and will continue to change rapidly, and the people are getting smarter the world over. As a result, organizations need to strategically change and adapt too. By using and adopting SWOT analysis, organizations can identify sources of competitive advantage and defeat and defuse threats by implementing strategic plans. This is what change is all about with implementation in place. This enables them to stay alive by achieving a sustainable profitability and business longevity in the global environment.

Chapter 3: Research Method

This study seeks to identify, describe, and analyze the state of health care in Nigeria, with primary research focus upon the city of Owerri and in the wider geographical area of Imo state. Since health care policy in Nigeria is marked by only a few published reports that may be valid in terms of current data, the proposed approach for this research is to use surveys, questionnaires, and interviews through which primary data can be obtained, along with an expansive review of corollary literature. Through this, tangible public policy models can be extracted and adapted for purposes of proposing a system for the design and delivery of cost effective and quality bases health care services in Owerri. During the research study, data collected through the research instruments, and information retrieved from the literature review will be analyzed and synthesized with the purpose of identifying evidence-based systemic gaps and formulating viable policy remedies.

Cooper and Schindler (2008) stated that the "main belief for performing essential qualitative research is to inquire and aim at achieving an in-depth understanding of a situation" (p. 162) of the investigator's interest as to provide and render a complete evaluation or analysis of the situation or phenomenon to be studied and gathering data which provide a detailed description of events or situations and interactions between people and things (pg 164) the action of knowledge is to verify and describe current state of affairs in the diagnosis, treatment, prevention of illness and disease and delivery of care (as in Owerri in Imo state of Nigeria). So understanding how to diagnose, treat and prevent ailment to the Owerri community, state of Imo and to produce a "HEALTHY" Nigeria becomes a major target and an essential planning dominant issue not only for Owerri alone but for both the state of Imo and Nigeria as a nation.

This research study will use a mixed research methodology where the qualitative and quantitative methods are applied. This is used and applied here to increase the perceived quality of the project. A qualitative strategy is aimed at analyzing existing information and data regarding government-ordained policies and practices that drive the current system of healthcare in Owerri and the state of Imo. An important advantage of the qualitative descriptive approach in the context of this study is that, by conducting a detailed review of the published literature, this approach offers the opportunity to capture a wide variety of issues, including low consumer expectations, a weak understanding of personal health, low life expectancy, ineffective and even erroneous diagnoses, lack of medicines, and outdated or non-existing medical equipment. Quantitative research method is the separation and conversion of data that is used to ensure that the problem statement and the research questions have been answered to the fullest possible degree. It tries to measure the situation of something by answering the questions related to how much, how often, how many, when, who or what is involved? This includes people or participants, questionnaires, and interview responses that are collected and extracted.

This research study has been conducted by using mainly the descriptive method, along with a quantitative and qualitative analysis approaches. Cooper and Schindler (2008) description of *descriptive research* can be summarized as a systematic discovery used to get data about issues or an issue, investigate condition, and analyze event or situation of what is at hand. That is to say, *what exists right here and now* that is important to the investigator within the issue, condition, event or situation at hand or phenomenon. Quantitative analysis will be used to deconstruct and interpret data, such as questionnaire responses, demographics, and health care indicators. Primary instrumentation will be composed of questionnaires and interviews. In addition, relevant case studies, policy reports, similar dissertations, and other published resources will be retrieved from a wide array of sources, including specialized online channels such as kwenu.com, Pub-Med, Motherland Nigeria and Search Nigeria.

During the research study, data collected through the research instruments, and information retrieved from the literature review will be analyzed and synthesized with the express purpose of enabling the researcher to identify evidence-based systemic gaps and to formulate viable policy remedies. Finally, quantitative decomposition of data will also be used to ensure that the problem statement and the research questions have been answered to the fullest possible degree.

Cooper and Schindler (2008) state that the main belief for performing essential research is to inquire and aim at achieving an in-depth understanding of a situation of the investigator's interest as to provide and render a complete evaluation or analysis of the situation or phenomenon, the action of knowledge is to verify and describe current state of affairs in the diagnosis, treatment, prevention of illness and disease and delivery of care in Owerri in Imo state of Nigeria. So understanding how to diagnose, treat and prevent ailment to make the Owerri community, state of Imo and a "HEALTHY" Nigeria becomes a major target and an essential planning dominant issue not only for Owerri alone but for both the state of Imo and Nigeria as a nation.

This research study will also use a qualitative strategy aimed at analyzing existing information and data regarding government-ordained policies and practices that drive the current system of healthcare in Owerri and the state of Imo. An important advantage of the qualitative descriptive approach in the context of this study is that, by conducting a detailed review of the published literature, this approach offers the opportunity to capture a wide variety of issues, including low consumer expectations, a weak understanding of personal health, low life expectancy, ineffective and even erroneous diagnoses, lack of medicines, and outdated or non-existing medical equipment.

The researcher and author of this study is an active and practicing Registered Nurse at Northeast Georgia Medical Center, Gainesville, Georgia, in the United States. The researcher is also a native of Owerri, with deep family ties in the area, and a strong understanding of local health care matters. In large part, the author's motivation for this research study is driven by personal and professional experiences in relation to health care in Owerri, and a keen sense of patriotism for the area and the country of Nigeria.

Methodology

This research study has been conducted by using mainly the descriptive method, along with a quantitative and qualitative analysis approaches. Cooper and Schindler (2008) description of *Descriptive Research* can be summarized as a systematic discovery used to get data about issues or an issue, investigate condition, and analyze event or situation of what is at hand. Quantitative analysis will be used to deconstruct and interpret data, such as questionnaire responses, demographics, and health care indicators. Primary instrumentation will be composed of questionnaires and interviews. In addition, relevant case studies, policy reports, similar dissertations, and other published resources will be retrieved from a wide array of sources, including specialized online channels such as kwenu.com, Pub-Med, Motherland Nigeria, and Search Nigeria.

During the research study, data collected through the research instruments, and information retrieved from the literature review will be analyzed and synthesized with the express purpose of enabling the researcher to identify evidence-based systemic gaps and to formulate viable policy remedies. Finally, quantitative decomposition of data will also be used to ensure that the problem statement and the research questions have been answered to the fullest possible degree.

Cooper and Schindler (2008) state that the main belief for performing essential research is to inquire and aim at achieving an in-depth understanding of a situation of the investigator's interest as to provide and render a complete evaluation or analysis of the situation or phenomenon... the action of knowledge is to verify and describe current state of affairs in the diagnosis, treatment, prevention of illness and disease and delivery of care in Owerri in Imo state of Nigeria. So understanding how to diagnose, treat and prevent ailment to make the Owerri community, state of Imo and a "HEALTHY" Nigeria becomes a major target and an essential planning dominant issue not only for Owerri alone but for both the state of Imo and Nigeria as a nation.

This research study will also use a qualitative strategy aimed at analyzing existing information and data regarding government-ordained policies and practices that drive the current system of healthcare in Owerri and the state of Imo. An important advantage of the qualitative descriptive approach in the context of this study is that, by conducting a detailed review of the published literature, this approach offers the opportunity to capture a wide variety of issues, including low consumer expectations, a weak understanding of personal health, low life expectancy, ineffective and even erroneous diagnoses, lack of medicines, and outdated or non-existing medical equipment.

The researcher and author of this study is an active and practicing Registered Nurse at Northeast Georgia Medical Center, Gainesville, Georgia, in the United States. The researcher is also a native of Owerri, with deep family ties in the area, and a strong understanding of local health care matters. In large part, the author's motivation for this research study is driven by personal and professional experiences in relation to health care in Owerri, and a keen sense of patriotism for the area and the country of Nigeria.

Research Questions

The research questions that guided this study were:

Research Question 1: How can health care delivery in Owerri be modified as to meet market and social demands?

Research Question 2: What kinds of policy recommendations may help alleviate the problem of care delivery in Owerri?

Instrumentation

A thorough and comprehensive review of related literature showed no existing document prior exists in the Owerri health care sector. This offered a satisfactory promise and encouragement to move forward with the particular objectives of this study. Primary data was collected through interviews and surveys. A questionnaire format was devised, and distributed to the selected participants. Secondary data were obtained through the review of published reports, studies, books, and other resources that are available online and in printed form.

Population and Sample

The target population of this study was defined as all employees and family members of employees over the age of eighteen (18) years of age or older. This participating population consists of students (part and full), non-students, teachers, civil servants, college professors, contract employees, family members and government officials. The sampling frame consists of universities that are coeducational, 15 health centers, 17 General Hospitals, 1 Teaching Hospital (State Economic and Empowerment and Development Strategy, 2004). A sample of 150 participants from the representative population was selected for the study. The 150 participants were comprised of adults over 18 years of age that work or reside in the area. Painstaking efforts have been made to obtain and ensure equitable representation of students of each gender. For this sample, random sampling was based on a sample interval of 20 participants.

Simple random sampling is a simple method that is used by the researcher to help choose and select units from the population the researcher is working with or interested in studying (in this case Owerri). Collectively the units form the sample size that the researcher is working with which is part of the larger number (the population) in this case, the Owerri people that the researcher is studying (like the 118 participants in the survey that are part of the larger (Owerri) population. This is important to the researcher as it is used to make estimated (statistical) inference about the larger population, achieve a representative sample of the population, for making good estimation (probability) selection, and for minimizing sampling bias or error.

Therefore, choosing or selecting the sample size was done by selecting the 150 units as the standard sample size made up of the 118 respondents as the unit members. The 150 representative as the sample size has an equal chance of being picked from the group or the (Owerri) population impacted by the poor health care service. These people are the units from the 150 sampled people, while the Owerri people (collectively) is the population represented by the small size or sample size of 150 people. So the 150 people were chosen from the Owerri population as a sample which became (or is) the sample size of 150 participants or units. This sample size was chosen because is a representation of the actual Owerri population.

Participation Selection

Participants are adults 18 years of age or older. All participants received basic instructions about the study knowing that the information is confidential and that they are protected from any harm. They also understand that the information is voluntary and benefit includes using the result to improve the health care service delivery in Owerri. Consent approval for the implementation of the study was obtained from participants freely and willingly.

The Procedure

Participants were asked to complete the questionnaires following consent and receiving the survey instructions. Each participant is handed over the cover letter (Appendix A) and questionnaire (Appendix B). In addition, participants also received brief verbal overview of the research project and instructed on proper research completion technique. Participants are then left alone, individually in the classroom for privacy and anonymity in the survey completion. After completion of the survey, participants exited the room through the exit door while placing the completed survey on the table by the exit door or anonymously leaving face down on the desk when done and leave. The participants completed the survey only once, as there was no opportunity for multiple completions.

Data Collection

The geographical locus of this research study has been the city of Owerri, located in the state of Imo in Nigeria. The city was formerly known as Owerri Local Government Area. Today, the city is comprised of Owerri Municipal, Owerri West, Owerri North and Ngor - Okpala (State Economic and Empowerment and Development Strategy, 2004). The research project will focus upon healthcare providers located in the old Owerri Local Government Area or just "Owerri or City of Owerri".

It consists of four main local government areas including Owerri Municipal, Owerri North and Owerri West and Ngor-Okpala with an estimated population of about 400,000 as of 2006. The local language is Igbo. Historically, it came into focus in the colonial era as an administrative capital of old Owerri province that stretched further to Umuahia and Port-Harcourt in the region. Meanwhile, Owerri is the Imo State capital city and the official administrative seat of the government. The city was plated by a team of designers from Switzerland in 1976 after its creation in February of 1976. It is one of the five major Igbo speaking cities in the southeastern region of the country of Nigeria. It is also a *passing city* to other nearby different southern states of Nigeria such as Rivers, Cross River, Bayelsa, Anambra and Abia. The inhabitants are mixed, made up primarily of indigenous and non-indigenous who work in public and private organizations in the area.

Data Analysis

Data collected in this study is descriptive in nature and was analyzed using descriptive technique. Part 1: The variables gender, marital status, number of children, health insurance coverage, employment status, level of satisfaction with private care physician (PCP), preferred health care facility and why go there, payment type, level of education, etc. were summarized using frequency and percentages in each category.

Part 2 is also descriptive in nature and was analyzed through summation and interval level variables. Participants were asked to indicate their degree of agreement or disagreement with a statement regarding the importance of free care in Owerri by choosing the right option to indicate "very important", "not very important"," not important", "undecided". Responses were then tallied and number of responses computed in percentages and interpreted, and represented in graphics (Chapter 4).

Human Participants and Ethics Precautions

All participants received an informed consent form. The use of signature and oral agreements removed the need for a separate consent form while ensuring each survey corresponds to an easily completed consent form. All participants obtained the proper e-mail and a phone number allowing them to ask questions at any time during the survey process and to view the results of the inquiry. The data remained anonymous, contained no identifying marks related to the participant, and could not be linked to institutions, participants, or collaborative efforts. No contact information, name, e-mail address, or other identification marks remained in a publicly accessible format. Likewise, no identifying phrases or terminologies from inquires remained in the data to ensure privacy during the feedback process.

Summary

The researcher discovered that the impact of revenue generation or funding by the state and federal governments for the development of the local government areas is lacking which has resulted in poor delivery, lack of staff motivation, bad road networks and transportation and poor development of the rural areas. Due to poor revenue generation to provide basic social amenities, such as access roads, schools, portable pipe-borne water, electricity among others it was impossible or difficult for rural people to sell their agricultural crops, drink portable water, or pay school fees. Thus, the poverty is very high and continuous. The researcher also discovered that due to poor revenue generation to provide basic social amenities especially in the rural areas, there is exodus of rural dwellers to the urban centers. Included in the researcher's findings was that the major method to be adopted by the local governments in order to improve revenue generation base should be the enlightenment of the citizens on the need and importance of regular payment of taxes.

Apart from these challenges there are other discovered unmet issues. Some of these include problems on transparency and accountability in the health care service delivery process that surfaced and are difficulty and problematic to fix. The sub-effect of all this is that of increasing corruption and malpractices in health service sector which has minimized the easy access for the public to health care services. In overall, this situation had made and lead the way to favoritism and nepotism, influences, kickbacks and improper gifts and gestures in delivering health services to the population more difficulty and essentially so. Overcoming these challenges is crucial in moving forward and to ensure a better health care service delivery system at the grassroots level. Following the researcher's recommendations is essential and will be helpful in overcoming these challenges and propelling health care services delivery forward in the area.

Chapter 4: Findings and Results

This section is concerned with the summation of the information process of the investigation. In presenting the information collected, separation of information is used to better interpret and understand the information received. The simple statistic method of frequencies and percentages have been used or applied in the process of analyzing the questionnaires.

Response Rate

There were 150 questionnaires issued for the study. Of the 150 issued, 118 were returned and 32 remained missing.

Demographic Data

The study measured several demographic variables and reports them along several dimensions.

Age

All respondents are of legal age and adults. For the purpose of presentation of the data, the author uses the number of completed questionnaires received back which is 118.

Gender

Of the respondents, 58% of the respondents were male and 42% of the respondents were female.

Live Alone Measure

Of the respondents, 28.8% lived alone while 71.2% lived with another person.

Marital Status

Of the respondents, 42.9% were single, 50% were married, and 0.2% was neither single nor married.

Children

Of the respondents, 49.2 % had children, 39.8% did not have children, and 11% neither want nor have children.

Personal Health

Of the respondents, 70% of the respondents believed to be in good health, 3% believed to be sick, 9% in fair health, while 2% was in bad or poor health. Approximately 16% was reported neither good or poor health.

Residency

Of the respondents, 89% were residents of Owerri local government area. About 7% are those were from other local government areas that live, attend school, or work in Owerri. The remaining 4% neither work nor live in Owerri.

Frequency of Check-Ups

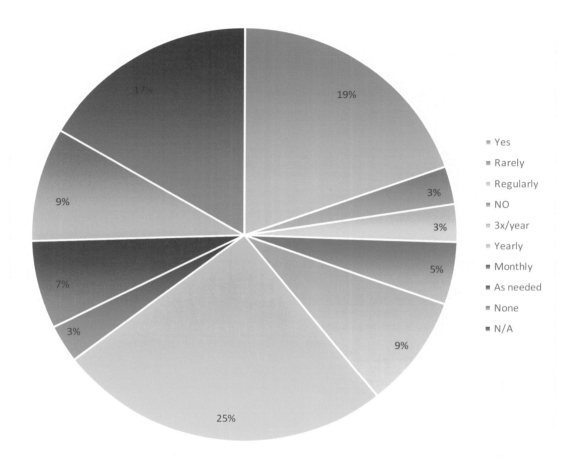

Legend:
- Yes
- Rarely
- Regularly
- NO
- 3x/year
- Yearly
- Monthly
- As needed
- None
- N/A

Figure 3. Frequency of check-ups reported by participants.

Figure 3 shows how poorly people manage their health and health problems by not going for frequent check-ups. It is clear and can be seen that regular scheduled medical check-up is out of the question here. Of the respondents, 12 or 10% of the respondents go for check-up twice a year, 20 or 17% go three times a year, 5 or 4% go five times a year, 14 respondents or 12% when sick, 10 or 8% go regularly (on schedule), 23 or 20% go as go as needed, 3 respondents or 3% go frequently (undefined), 6 or 5% of the respondents as not all, 6 or 5% for yearly check-ups and 19 or 16% of the respondents as not applicable. This in general explains why and how lack of regular check-ups can lead to prevalence of complex emergencies and chronic conditions among the people that would have been otherwise prevented. It becomes important to educate the public about the long term impact, importance and effect of regular and routine check-ups with their doctors. By so doing, simple problems that could become big ones latter can be detected early and treated while complex ones are evaluated and properly managed.

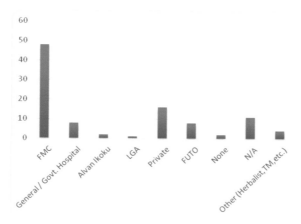

Figure 4. Hospital use as reported by participants.

Figure 4 shows information and attendance preference of people and the hospitals they use for treatment are not by choice or like pattern rather as a matter of "Can't help, lack of choice, or urgency". The Federal Medical Center (FMC), Owerri and the private-patented medicine took the leads here. For FMC, this is true because the respondents believe it has more amenities than others as a federal institution, while the private-patented medicine has the convenience of "in and out" service to the patients and customers as noted by the respondents.

Approval Ratings of FMC

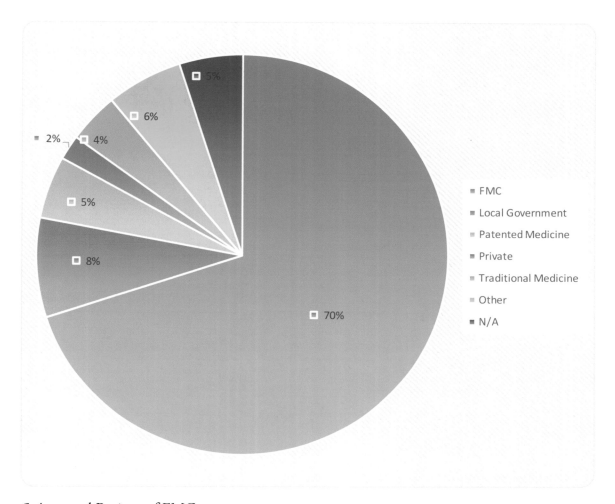

Figure 5. Approval Ratings of FMC.

From figure 5, 83 or 70% of the people out of the total of 118 believe going to FMC is the best thing not only because is a federal institution with more amenities but because the evaluation is better with more specialists than others. This is why they prefer to go there. Secondly, those who go to Local Government Hospitals say they do so because they are cheaper and more affordable than the FMC. This is wrong and should not be so because it sends the wrong message. Citizens should not hold their health hostage just to trade their life for cheap service because of affordability. The Federal Government can step up in this regard. Other sources such as mobilizing and using the public resources with their philanthropists and foreign aid can be tapped to alleviate this problem. This is why citizens resort to traditional Medicine as an option that may not be appropriate.

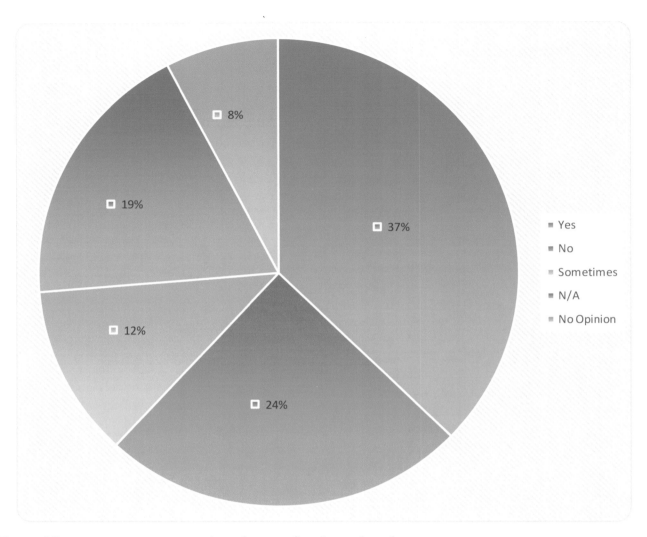

Figure 6. Participant opinion regarding the use of traditional medicine.

According to Young's Choice Making Model (1981), a sick person will not use or refuse treatment if they feels it will not work, or not accessible. Being accessible means examining the total treatment (service) expenses and how the price will match the treatment or service needed i.e. an evaluation of the process. This, which when lacking (as in the case of Owerri) may convince people to try and use the home or traditional remedy they know or deem possible which may not be right or appropriate for the condition as an option.

Distance from Hospital

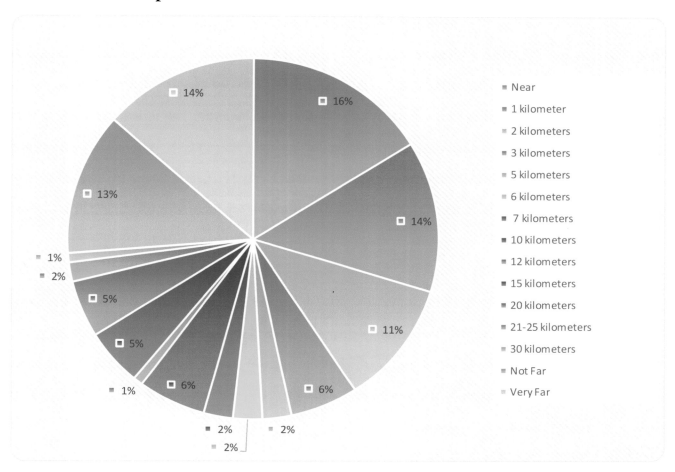

Figure 7. Distances between hospital and customer.

Figure 7 shows the impact of distance on health care service in Owerri. It can be stated that the nearer the distance, the more the utilization while "Very Far" indicates the opposite in terms of transportation, access, utilization and overall cost.

PCP Opinions

Of the respondents, 58 or 49% of the respondents have PCP while nearly same number, 56 or 48% have none and 4 or 3% is not applicable or have no opinion regarding PCP. This undercuts the benefits of patient-doctor relationship. Visiting the doctor only when sick or as needed basis is a disservice to the patient population as more preventable ailments such as hypertension or diabetes, etc. can be detected early, treated and managed through routine doctor's visit rather than waiting and going when is too late, too complex and advanced in the game that can have or result in a negative outcome. Furthermore, having a PCP helps establish a baseline early enough for the patient that can help the doctor evaluate patient as or when needed as the case may be.

Medical Doctor Specialty

Of the respondents, only 12 respondents or 10% of the 118 respondents say their doctor is internal medicine, 8 or 7% is neurology, 3 or 3% is cardiovascular, 4 or 3% is orthopedics, 45 or 38% is general practice, 30 or 25% don't know and 16 or 14% is not applicable. This data show the need for increase in healthcare specialization with special interest in MD specialties in addition to communicating and educating the patients about their specialties, interests and their clients' health.

Medical Doctor Satisfaction Rates

Of the respondents, only 36% of the respondents say they are very satisfied with their doctors, while 32% of them say they are satisfied. Only about 8% of the people say they are averagely satisfied, 12% unsatisfied, while the other 12% say it does not matter or have no opinion.

Transportation to the Medical Doctor

Of the respondents, 34 respondents or 29% of those surveyed use public transport for their medical appointments while 49 or 42% of them have no opinion or it does not matter. For 1.21B, 114 or 97% of the 118 respondent said the government does not provide any kind of transportation for either the doctor or hospital visit. This could be expensive as a factor affecting health service utilization. We can now see why the citizens of Owerri would either prefer to look for a nearby facility or a cheaper treatment alternative due to transportation difficulty which affects access; hence the traditional medicine (TM) as an option. As a result, they have to find a way to get to the hospital or to their doctors only when sick and not for routine check-up individually on their own. Therefore, some kind of ride or transportation assistance can alleviate this problem.

Transportation Refunds

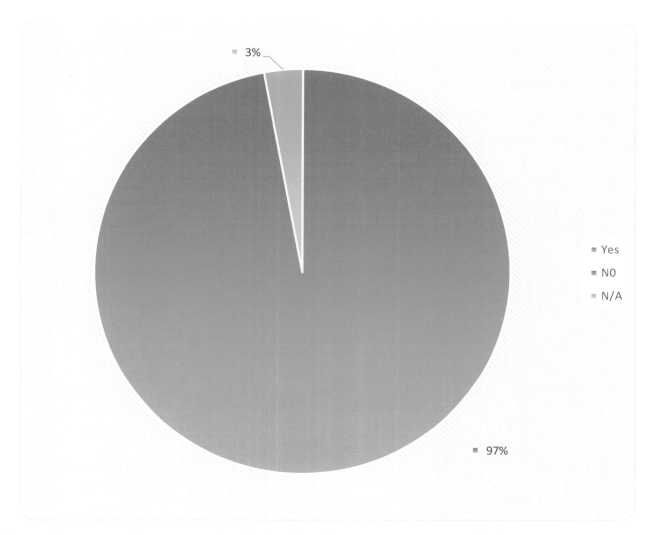

Figure 8. Percentage of participants by whether they obtain a transportation refund.

Figure 8 shows that personal expenses can affect health care service and utilization for the citizens. Therefore, finding a cheaper health care option such as traditional medicine becomes the only alternative for most of the people in treating their ailments which can also affect outcome as a result of this kind of "junk medicine or quarks".

Being Prevented from Visiting the Medical Doctor

Of the respondents, 41% cited money or cost related issues or expenses as a major factor preventing them from going to the doctor or seeking medical help, while 14% neither care nor have an opinion about it. Also 10 (8%) out of the 118 respondents cited work as a reason for not seeing the doctor while 10 or 8% of the respondent cited their reason as being sick, while 9 or 8% indicated lack of transportation as their main reason.

This goes to buttress the effect of good road and adequate transportation as major factors to healthcare service delivery particularly in the area. It is also worthy to observe that 7% of the respondents indicated needless going to the doctor since they are not sick forgetting that prevention is better than cure and this is a known fact and also indicating lack of education and understanding of real or true health. This is like time bomb waiting to explode out of pure ignorance.

Reason for Previous Medical Visit

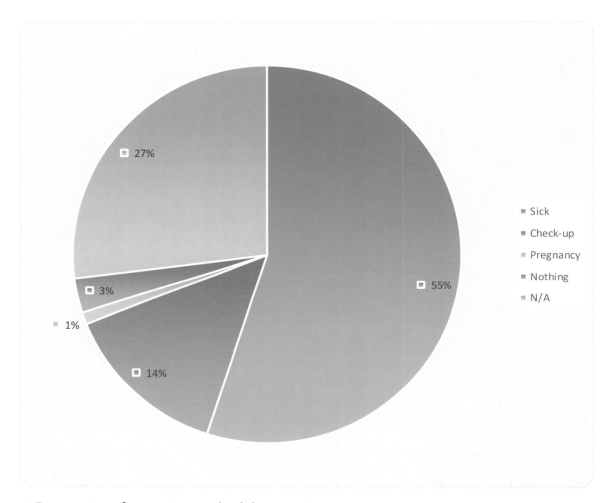

Figure 9. Reason given for previous medical doctor visit.

Of the respondents, 55% visit the doctor or seek medical attention only when they are sick rather than maintaining routine or regular check–ups for prevention as noted earlier. It is also noted that only 14% of them go for check–ups while 27% do not care or have no opinion about it.

Diagnostic Reason for Previous Visit

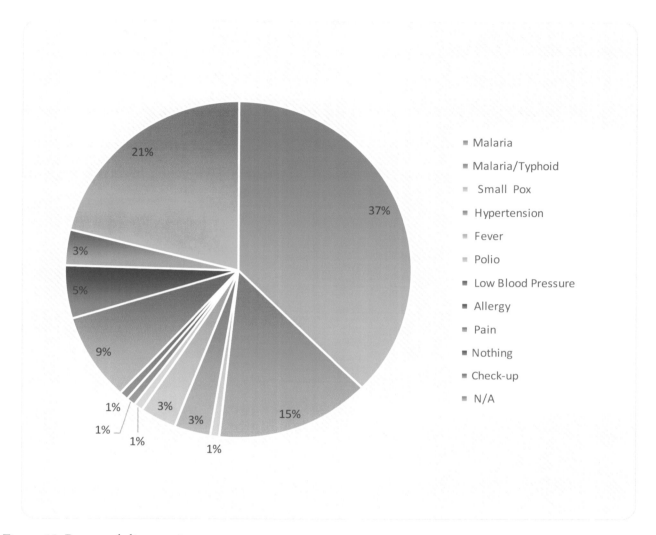

Figure 10. Reported diagnostic reasons.

Of the respondents, 37% of the respondents suffered malaria while 15 % of them suffered from Malaria and typhoid. Apart from anything else, these are preventable conditions including small pox, polio, fever, and pain, while 21% of them have no opinion or not applicable on the issue. As a result, these can be attributed to poor health maintenance, lack of enlightenment or public education and inadequate understanding of common ailment preventive measures in the area (if not statewide or even national).

Participants Worried about Healthcare in Owerri

Of the respondents, 80% indicated worried about the health care in Owerri, while 20 or 17% of them feel the opposite and 4 or 3% has no opinion or do not care. This shows and means that the current health care system does not meet the needs of the people, hence the study for a new approach to the problem. This is extremely important for the leadership to note and understand the feelings, opinion and the wishes of the people they serve for what they are saying for a change or the ability to do better.

Foreign Charity in Owerri

Of the respondents, 85% approved to see some kind of charity involvement in the Owerri healthcare delivery system for a change, while 8 or 7% of the respondents disapprove and 10 or 8% of the respondents do not care or have no opinion at all in the matter. This case is an observable fact as the majority of the people want to see some change or improvement in the healthcare system in Owerri and Imo State that was also referenced above in Question 1.26.

Free Health Care in Owerri

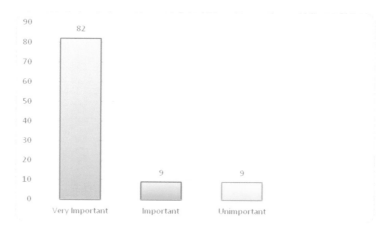

Figure 11. Free health care in Owerri.

Of the respondents, 82% indicated approval for free healthcare in Owerri while 11 or 9% of them feel is not important or disapproval and approximately 9% or 10 respondents think the issue is unimportant.

Participants Have Healthcare Insurance in Owerri

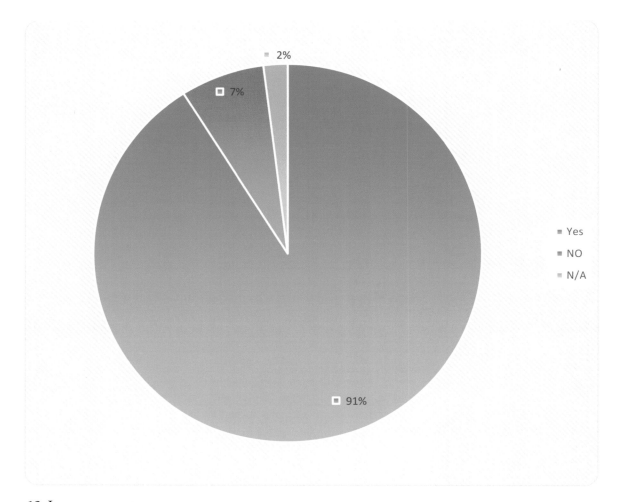

Figure 12. Insurance coverage.

It is clear that the citizens of Owerri want some form of health insurance coverage for their health service. As noted from the above, 108 of the 118 respondents or approximately 91% want some form of insurance coverage while 8 or 7% of the respondents say no and 2 or approximately 2% of them do not care or have no opinion.

Participants Pay Little Money to Improve Healthcare Service

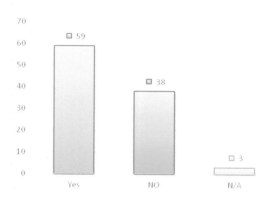

Figure 13. Participant willingness to pay into healthcare improvements.

Of the respondents, 59% of those surveyed indicated willingness to pay a little or some form of money to support and improve the healthcare service system in Owerri. In addition, 45 or 38% of them disapprove the idea while 3 or approximately 3% of the respondents neither approve nor disapprove the idea as noted. This shows that some of the participants understand the importance of coverage and that it will be wise to pay a little to subsidize the cost thereby helping for the underprivileged.

Current Employment

It can be ascertained that unemployment is equally an added problem to healthcare issues. While 60 or 51% of the 118 respondents is unemployed, only 58 out of 118 or 49% is employed. This is an economic loss that can put additional burden on the system with already limited resources stretched as it is.

Current Employer

Of the respondents, 47 % work for the ministry as the major employer, while 33 or 28% of the respondents work in the private sector and 16 or 14% of the respondents has no work, and 13 or 11% of the respondents with neither job nor opinion.

Type of Employment

In explaining the information, 42 or 36 % of the respondents are management staff, while 52 or 44% of them are non-management staff. So, while 44% of the respondents are non-management staff, 24 or 20% of them are either no management or not working at all.

Medical Expenses in Thousands of Naira

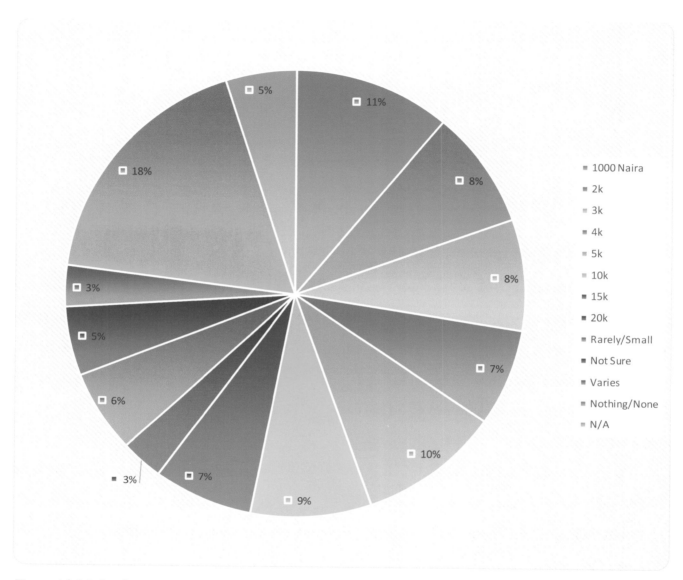

Figure 14. Medical expenses.

It is clear that the medical spending is not commensurate with income.

Medical Insurance

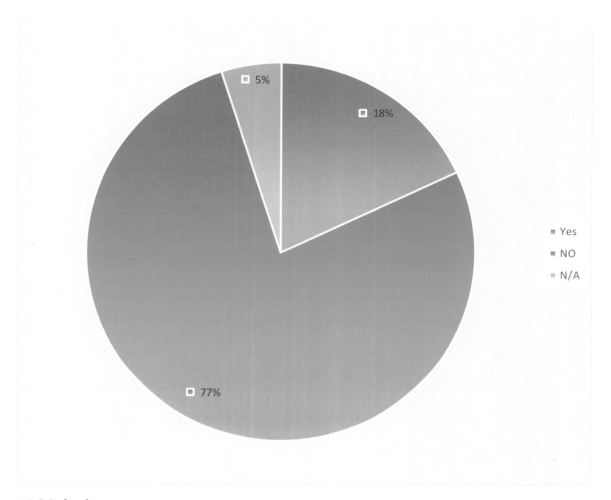

Figure 15. Medical insurance percentages.

Of the respondents, 77% of the respondents say "NO" to medical insurance while 18% say "Yes" and 5% is not applicable or do not care. This primarily reflects the opinion of management staff who probably can afford to pay for their own medical services versus question 1.32 where majority of the ordinary working people (91%) want some form of insurance coverage.

Employer Provided Coverage

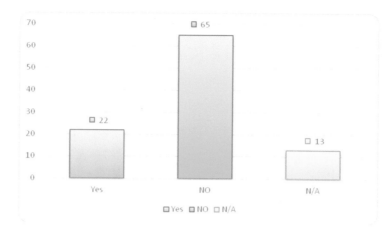

Figure 15. Employer provided coverage.

There is the need for improvement in this area of healthcare coverage. Hopefully, it will be universal such that employer pays it or some proportion of it for all across the board.

Types of Coverage

While 20 or 17% of the respondents are family, 15 or 13% of the respondents is individual. In addition, while 39 or 33% of the respondents has neither family nor individual coverage, 44 or 37% of the respondents has neither coverage nor opinion about insurance coverage.

Employer Contribution to Insurance

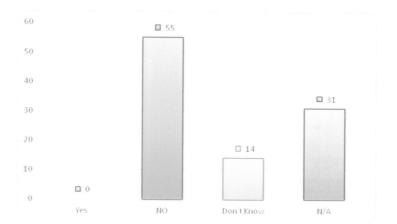

Figure 16. Employer contributions.

It is clear that employer pays or makes no contribution whatsoever toward medical insurance coverage for their employees. While 65 or 55% of the respondents say no employer insurance coverage or contribution, 16 or 14% of the respondents do not know while 37 or 31% has no opinion to the situation.

Employer Pays Insurance or Medical Expense Refund

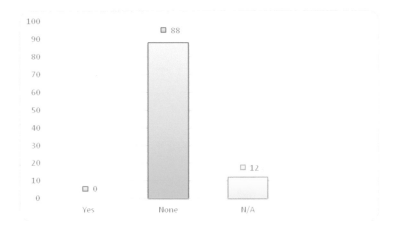

Figure 17. Refund rates.

Of the respondents, 88% no employer insurance contribution and 14 or 12% of them agreed nor have no opinion. Therefore, it is very true that most of the respondents agree that employer do not pay or contribute for insurance coverage or payment in any way or form.

Compensation

It can be said that the number of wage earners decreases as compensation increases rather than the opposite; hence 8% earns less than 20,000 Naira, while only 3% earns 91-100 thousand and 4% greater than 101 thousand. This may be related to educational background or any other compensation qualification criteria obtainable in the area.

Concerns Regarding Healthcare

Approximately 70% of the respondents say they are worried or concerned about the healthcare system in Owerri, while 27 or 23% say no, and 8 or 7% of them say not applicable or have no opinion.

Worried About Healthcare

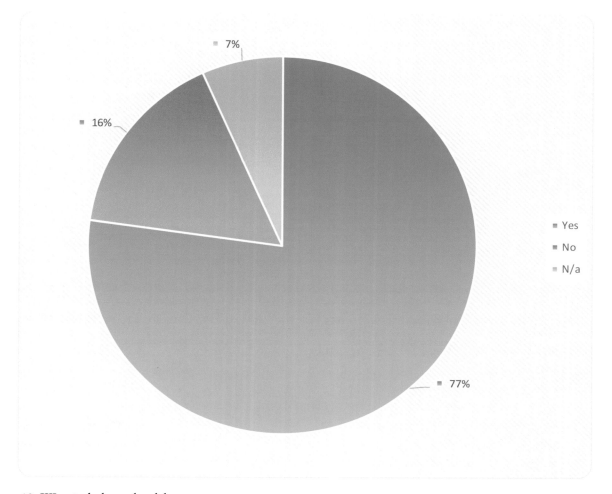

Figure 18. Worried about health care.

In general terms, people are concerned about their healthcare and the message is clear. The question here is whether the government is willing and ready to listen to the voice of the people is a different matter altogether. This is a change we all must collectively fight for in good faith.

Free Health Care in Imo State

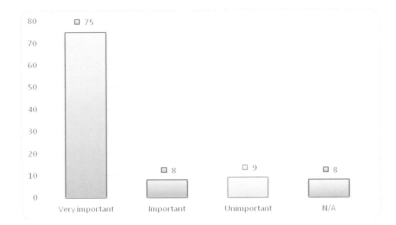

Figure 19. Free health care in Imo State

Approximately 75% of the respondents expressed concern about the healthcare system in the state. This reflects the response for the Owerri area that is crucial for the local leaders, the state and national representatives and their policy agenda at different levels respectively.

Pay Little to No Money to Support the System

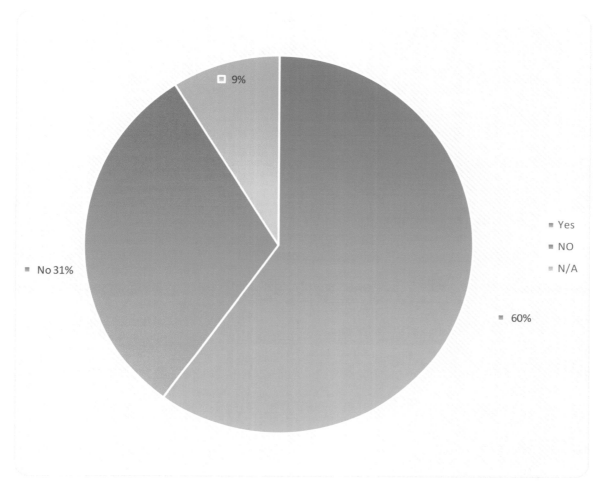

Figure 20. Pay little to no money to support the system.

Of the respondents, 60% of the respondents would like to pay some money (at least 5%) to support the healthcare system in Owerri or the state of Imo. This is not a bad idea in terms of policy so that the government can have some revenue from the citizens to put toward the project with all good intention.

Foreign Charities in Imo State

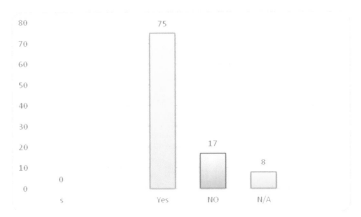

Figure 21. Foreign charities in Imo State.

About 75% of the respondents want foreign charities in Owerri and Imo state. This they believe will help fill the existing gaps in skilled manpower, supply equipment, offer training, better management and address policy issues.

Male and Female Employment Compensation

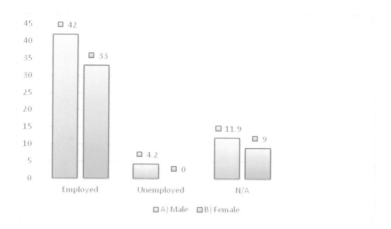

Figure 22. Male and female employment compensation.

Male employment compensation. Of the respondents, 69 male respondents only 64 of them are gainfully employed. Out of this number, 50 of them or 42.4% receive compensation while 14 or 11.9% do not, may be retired, not available, disabled due to poor health or maintenance, etc.

Female employment compensation. Of the respondents, only 33% of them are employed. Among the 49 respondents, only 10 or 9% of them are unemployed i.e. do not receive any kind of payment or salary for their service, not available, retired or disable due to poor health or maintenance.

FRN Analyis

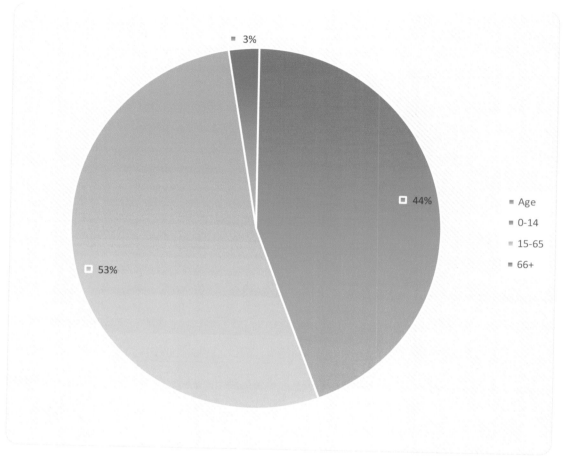

Figure 23. FRN analysis.

Figure 23 confirms the employment data in this study above. That is to say, above 65 years of age manpower begins to dwindle, strangled, lacking or even non-existent. The study data suggest that either this age retires early due to poor health or health care management and maintenance related issues or completely displaced by the younger generation and out of the manpower market completely, thus, creating room for the younger ones. This is an economic waste that could be costly. In general, the best solution here as noted earlier is the implementation of better health care policies that can attend to the needs of the citizens by answering their health care calls of all particularly with this age group inclusive.

Findings

Above all, this project examined and discussed the hope surrounding the Owerri health care service to the people. It showed how and why gaps existed and how different governments failed the people in providing adequate and affordable healthcare for the population. The paper makes a contribution by sending messages to the government and representatives alike for understanding the expectations of the people regarding health care. Findings are provided in this project so that they can be applied and adapted to improve and facilitate the delivery of health care service in the area. This section is concerned with the summation of the information process of the investigation. In presenting the information collected, separation of information is used to better interpret and understand the information received. The simple statistic method of frequencies and percentages have been used or applied in the process of analyzing the questionnaires.

In this analysis, the researcher presented a summary of the findings based on the analysis of the data collected. The findings of this study is that Local Government Areas do not have an appropriate constitutional and legal framework, institutional capacity, service delivery mechanism built in by public-private partnership and mutual understanding between national and local political leadership to get the job done for the people in the area. These situations contributed to the emergence of the various challenges facing health care service delivery system in the area as noted and investigated through questionnaires and interviews of the study

Summary

There is the need for doing better with the existing hospitals and other providers in the area. Undoubtedly, there is no doubt that patented medicine has a role to play in fulfilling the medical needs of the people including the significance of traditional medicine. But it is understandable that its role in terms of diagnosis and treatment options is limited. The benefits of quick and easy convenient service of available medications are there to stay better than the hospital organization. There is the need for more and better hospital system both in Owerri and Imo State because the Federal Medical Center (FMC) cannot solve the entire medical needs of the people or else it will run out of gas over time. There is an urgent need for more and better equipped hospitals in Owerri as well as the state. May be the government can contract with private organizations to improve the already existing substandard facilities for better operations rather than mushrooming mediocre facilities and organizations that are up to no good. Private bids can be sort in a cooperative manner or these substandard facilities auctioned out to make room for a much better functioning and equipped and updated ones that can serve the people well.

Chapter 5: Summary, Conclusions, and Recommendations

Introduction

In investigating the Owerri healthcare service delivery situation, this study aims at exploring the challenges of the local government healthcare service delivery in Owerri, Imo State of Nigeria. In view of this, Owerri and its newly constituted LGAs were selected as a case study. Through this case study, the researcher tries to find the answers to the research questions of what are the challenges faced by the LGAs in terms of better health care service delivery for the area. And how the LGAs would overcome these challenges and what innovations and strategies would work in delivering a better health care service to the people remains the focus. The study also tested hypothesis of constitutional and legal framework, consistency politics, institutional capacity and service delivery mechanism built up by public-private partnership at the micro level that can ensure a better health care service delivery for the people of the area.

Summary

This study was largely guided by the service delivery models especially decentralization of service delivery model and alternative service delivery model (multi-level governance model). These models identified the following as crucial variables affecting the better service delivery at the lower levels of government:

- Lack of constitutional and legal framework,
- Lack of consistency politics,
- Lack of institutional capacity to do the job, and
- Lack of built-in service delivery mechanism or initiative.

Taking these variables into consideration, analytical framework has been developed. This framework analyzes what are the challenges faced by Owerri and its LGAs in terms of better healthcare service delivery. And how the LGAs would overcome these challenges and what innovations and strategies would work for delivering the badly needed healthcare services to the population as indicated by the findings remains to be seen.

Conclusions

In conclusion, the cost of poor quality health care service delivery in the health care sector includes loss of lives, loss of public confidence, low staff morale, and wastage of limited resources to say the least. Therefore, with this in mind, let us not make the health care service delivery and utilization a policy of the celebration of words and exaggeration of position of power. The governments have to be engaged with the people and their health care needs. According to the United Nations Organization (2003), health care is a fundamental human rights that must be upheld, supported, and sustained through policy initiatives that should have the best interest of the citizens at heart. So let us get to work for the interest of the people (not personal). From this research, it is clear that poor health care delivery cannot be tolerated by the population any longer. The rural political areas and their leadership for better planning should develop a method of action for the purpose of directing and conducting quality service for the people. This is crucial for the interest of all. Therefore, the local government areas and their management should strategically plan on proper measures to conduct their service, functions and responsibilities to meet the needs of the people as provided by the constitution of the country.

Discussion
Difficulties in Undertaking the Health Service Delivery In Owerri

One of the major challenges faced by the health care services delivery sector in Owerri is that powers and functions assigned through section 40 of the Municipal Council Ordinance have not been clearly defined and according to provision of the thirteenth Amendment to the Nigerian constitution by the Abacha administration (1987). Such powers and functions are expected to be exercised under the control of the Nigerian Constitution. But powers and functions of a local government institution should be clearly defined (as it constitutes the weakest tier of government in the federal system) through an appropriate constitutional and legal framework. Through this process, central government (such as Nigerian Government) must be willing to give up control and recognize the importance of sub-national government in service delivery. Legal powers in recruiting needed staff to the Local Government Area council have been assigned to Local Government Area Council under the provision of Local Government Area Ordinance and under the amendment to the constitution. As the power of recruiting staff has been assigned to two institutions, it has complicated the situation to filling vacancies of posts of vocational and technological experts who are playing a major role in delivering health services.

As well, power of taking actions regarding removing unauthorized buildings and against business places that could be a threat to health and sanitation has also been given to Local Government through the Municipal Council ordinance. But the Central Government has also assigned this power to other Statutory Boards and Authorities to the LGA. The end result of assigning some powers to two institutions is increasing conflicts between the two institutions regarding exercising such powers. Interviews held with some management staff further proved this situation. The Owerri LGA Council has been given some power and functions regarding delivery of health services under LGA Council Ordinance. But when exercises are started, such powers (have to) face some problems with the State Government. The end result of that conflict is that State government delays or decreases their funds to LGAs or just dead on arrival. The simple truth is that this should not be so, but it is.

In addition, the political powers that were used to promote disease free environment and sanitation of the municipal areas are not utilized with the objective of better health service delivery. For instance, even though medical and health officials have been assigned necessary powers to inspected and regularize dirty waste in Owerri, sometime this kind of power conflict do exist in the process of execution as noted by Uwadi (2011) in his article captioned " Owerri the dirtiest City in Nigeria" .

Encouraging Public Participation in the Owerri Healthcare Service Delivery

With the aim of mobilizing the public to participate in health care service delivery, this researcher shows and strongly makes the following additional recommendations regarding this proposed process:

- That the Owerri Municipal and the LGAs initiate various strategies such as the 'Citizens' Council', Chairman's Community Services Commission', 'The Public Mission Department' and 'Our Roads Task Force Management or Local Government Roads Commission' etc. Implementing programs such as these will give and create the opportunity for the public and private sectors to participate in decision making process, and decide the type of health and other basic social services they need and require. It also has an effect to enhance the cooperation and satisfaction level of the public on the current standards and quality of the health service delivery. This will help reestablish the eroded public trust and confidence in public service.

- In analyzing the health service delivery in Owerri, this study mainly found out that as a decentralized LG institution, the Owerri LGAs can introduce strategies and innovations that would developed partnership with the private sector and enhance public participation that can improve and better the health service delivery for the people. As a result of this, efficiency and effectiveness of delivering healthcare service will improve in the area. But, with the removal of all the political inconsistencies, the political administrative situations between national and local political leadership, the situation of things will hopefully improve at the local level.

- If the above mentioned strategies are paralyzed, and local communities had to face the numerous difficulties regarding the access to basic health services from the LGAs, the situation will result in decreasing efficiency and effectiveness of the delivering of health services. As a result, making the end result of the health care service delivery more complex and complicated. Therefore, the LGAs should implement the recommended strategies and to provide disease preventive services in order to keep the municipal areas as a sanitation zone avoiding the spread of contagious and epidemic diseases. AS a result, the implementation of these policies or programs will better the functioning of the governments which results in a better healthcare delivering system for the Owerri population.

Adopting the Health Care Service Excellence Model.

The health care Service Excellence Model is a service production concept that is research based service improvement and quality model that aims at improvement, competence, confidence and quality of service. It is offered and proposed as a solution to the lack of education and training or retraining of the Owerri healthcare staff. It has six components for enhancing and improving organizational output or bottom line through the collective collaboration of these components for improvement through education as noted here below. The Six Components of the Excellence Model are:

- Training and empowering of staff;
- Improving employee skills, job satisfaction and competence;
- Earning superior healthcare skills or service delivery;
- Improved healthcare service delivery and satisfaction;
- Improved (positive) customer service outcome and loyalty with and increased profit margin;
- Customer or patient loyalty and retention.

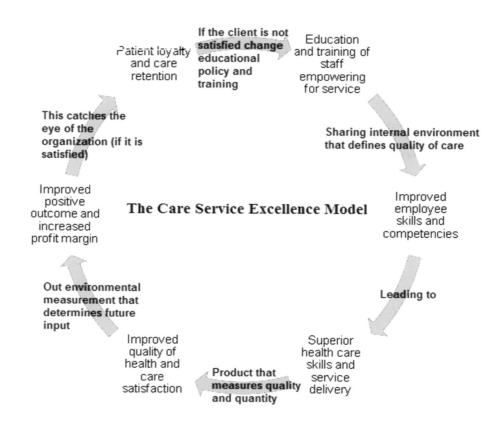

Figure 24. The Care Service Excellence Model.

Therefore, the Health Care Service Excellence Model (HCSEM) starts with educating and training of staff to be well prepared, positioned and empowered for service or organizational production of their product. Thus, thereby improving skills, confidence and competence, giving rise to excellent service delivery by improving employee (their) skills. By rendering quality or excellent care in this model, stakeholders, clients and families are happy and satisfied. This attitude is trusting and reassuring resulting in positive outcome and more client-family satisfaction. In addition, improved patient care or service leads to better client outcome and satisfaction thereby bringing about customer or patient loyalty, retention and relation, etc. The commonality here is that the model is also virtuous and circular in nature as seen in the diagram and also improves quality without limit.

As noted by Reichheld (2003), this model goes beyond customer and employees. Although there are other ways to arrive at the same or similar conclusion, but the major advantage of this expansion model is that is open and flexible thereby allowing anyone or organization to "do it their way". It also emphasizes the benefits of education and investing on employees by helping them reach their highest potential that can impact the overall outcome in the organizational bottom line. Hence, it shows the impact of educating, improving, investing, empowering staff and as well as believing in the organizational manpower for a better and quality outcome keeping in mind that change or improvement may not always happen by way of traditional method, or process but by innovation. Selecting, applying and expanding this model is also seen as an organizational process guide that can yield positive result in terms of investment, research and development. It also encourages and maintains customer and employee retention. It also ensures quality and reliable service relationship. It also standardizes and improves the service recipe process which is good news from the organizational point of view particularly in healthcare. Above all, it also has the advantage of internal service control and precision in the training and service processes leading to perfection.

In addition, the following are other healthcare factors noted to be affecting Owerri healthcare service sector as a whole that this model can also be of great help:

- High cost of service
- Lack of current health technological equipment
- Increase aging population
- Rural to urban migration
- Poor access to health service
- Poor or lack of good alternative medical therapy
- Poor lifestyle or lack of behavior changes
- Healthcare staff attitude or brush offs, runarounds, meanness, or coldness

Summary of the Findings

In the analysis of this study, the researcher presented a summary of the findings based on the analysis of the data collected. The findings of this study is that though as a decentralized local government institution, local government areas using and implementing these strategies and innovations will help themselves preplan, modify, and readjust by uniting and developing partnership with the private sector thereby enhancing the public participation in the health care service delivery process in the area of cooperation that failed in the past. This type of cooperative principle and teamwork help to ensure to pull off the health care service delivery and expansion to the people of Owerri. The main factor for this type of cooperative failure in the past is that the Local Government Areas do not have an appropriate constitutional and legal framework, institutional capacity, service delivery mechanism built in by public-private partnership and mutual understanding between national and local political leadership. These situations contributed to the emergence of the various challenges facing health care service delivery system in the area as noted below. These are:

Shortage of sufficient and competent human resources such as trained and skilled personnel for health care service delivery in Owerri.

Unclear powers and functions of the Local Government Areas to undertake the health care services delivery process.

- Poor public–private partnership and cooperation.
- Inadequate financial resources and funding of the health care sector.
- Lack of infrastructural provision such as facilities, adequate road network and other physical structures and resources, and inadequate maintenance thereafter.
- Lack of community access to health care services.
- Inconsistency of policies and politics.
- Inadequate health service and unqualified health care and medical personnel.
- Inadequate supply and maintenance of medical equipment and supplies
- Poor facility management and infrastructural maintenance
- Bad management, leadership and lack of commitment
- Lack of adequate monitoring and supervision of the management process
- Bad road network and lack of transportation for the population
- Lack of sustained power supply or electric generating equipment
- High medical and health care cost
- Lack of control and monitoring of fake drugs and quacks
- Callous attitude of the government officials and local representatives
- Lack of proper financial monitoring and supervision of the general spending (corruption)
- Lack of adequate education and training of the medical staff and continuing education thereafter
- Poor public interest and participation in government particularly matters affecting their lives
- Lack of transparency and accountability among government officials and local representatives (corruption)
- Increase in corruption such as mistrust, kickbacks and misappropriation of funds.

Recommendations

Based on these findings, the following recommendations or proposals have been made and following and implementing them will be helpful to overcoming these challenges. Because of the principal elements of these findings, the following proposals are put forward as accepted solutions to help overcome the Owerri health care challenges. These are:

- The exertion of power of the rural governments and their leaders should not only be aimed at revenue contributions alone but also to the supply of services devoted to the people living in the area such as hospitals, good access roads, power supply, running water supply and other living needs that can help improve or facilitate the life of the local communities and their families.

- Introduce market competition, use of email, electronic device, good healthcare policy such as patient rights and protection, and maintaining good medical records.

- Reduce and improve cost and production of medication and drugs.

- Invest in research and development for the health care sector through the institutions of higher learning by making grants and other funds available.

- Offer payment incentives to healthcare professionals in form of salary, education funding, scholarships—particularly in the rural suburbs for doctors, nurses and other allied health workers choosing to live and work in such rural areas. It will also be helpful to make their pay scale commensurate and competitive to that of the business world or the private sector.

- Increase admission to that of both nursing and medical schools to ensure availability of highly trained staff in all fields of healthcare and to keep abreast of the latest technological practices in the field and its services.

- Doctor partners: Apart from referrals, this is a systematic process where the doctors from the neighboring facilities and organizations partner together, share special equipment with one another and referring patients that need special care or evaluation to where is available particularly with FMC. That way patients can get quality care with proper or better outcome. Managing this kind of innovative network can make a big difference in the life of the population by improving health care service delivery, quality of care and improved health status or outcome.

- The government can provide and subsidize transportation for patients for this kind of treatment or referral to help alleviate the burden of cost and inconvenience for the citizens toward quality care particularly the old adult or the elderly and children.

- Inauguration and creation of Citizens' Referral Service: Inaugurating and creating citizens' or patients' referral service whose primary function is charged with the responsibility of assisting the citizens with the transportation program and keeping their medical appointments will not be a bad idea.

- Provision of more health care facilities in the local areas and communities and equip all to standard for convenience, efficiency and effectiveness.

- Create more awareness campaign on all health services particularly health promotion and disease prevention such as immunization, pre and post natal care, health/preventive screening, nutrition and environmental health, and promoting health education in elementary and secondary schools will not be a bad idea.

- The creation, development and implementation of comprehensive health care financing system particularly for the rural and urban poor should also be considered.

- Increase awareness of reproductive health education such as for HIV and AIDS and formulate adequate and properly appropriate policies that should always be reviewed, adapted and adopted with changing time of the future and beyond.

- Judiciously improve, adopt and implement adequate budget allocation to health care sector not only at the local level but also at both state and federal levels.

- In terms of health care service delivery in Owerri, the government should look to improving governance, personnel and leadership issues, create, use and take advantages of essential policies, rules and regulations that can benefit the people through the actions of the local leadership. This will help it to strive high to ensure improved access, quality and use of medical products and through technology.

- The Federal Government of Nigeria can enhance quality of care by providing adequate medical equipment and interactive computers (with programs) that can assist healthcare providers and professionals with decision making tasks and capabilities. Such will facilitate and solidify the move by funding to ensure that adequate staffing, equipment and health care infrastructures are properly supplied and facilities adequately equipped. This will help the healthcare professionals in fulfilling their fiduciary obligations (for their patients) for managing and evaluating their disease conditions. The fulfillment of this crucial role is currently lacking at all levels of government and administration.

- It will also be wise "to address the underlying social and economic issues and determinants of health (such as lifestyle) through policies and programs that enhance health equity and integrate pro-poor, gender-responsive, and human rights - based approaches". Second, is to promote a healthier environment, intensify primary prevention and influence public policies in all sectors so as to address the root causes of the environmental threats to health such as malaria that was earlier addressed.

- Establish some legislative action for free care especially for the disabled, the poor and the elderly in the area (or even within the state)

- Involve corporations and other private entities and organizations in the policy making process as shareholders

- Set up an inspectional body equivalent to that of the U.S Joint Commission for healthcare providers that can set general performance guidelines and organizational standards and monitor compliance of the organizations and health care facilities and providers statewide (which may and could also be a national model).

- Improve and provide technological equipment that can enable all doctors and other healthcare providers to share information and communicate necessary healthcare information that can appropriately benefit their patients and their families and other customers

- Provide more specialist hospitals with quality and qualified doctors, nurses and other professionals that can help evaluate, treat and manage the people's health.

- Provide mobile clinics and services that can help service the underprivileged particularly the disabled in the remote villages that has no means of transportation or access to healthcare as members of the society or community through the referral service (mentioned earlier No. 9)

- Increase and improve early public education in elementary and secondary schools on the advantages of preventive health (e.g. check ups, immunization, etc.) and early detection of health problems for convenience and efficiency

- Provide incentives for medical training and education of related fields particularly in city and state schools and universities. But until then, hire outside doctors, nurses, lab techs and other needed professionals to fill and service the existing hospitals and facilities to provide the immediate care needed by the citizens

- The government should also enact laws and policies that can increase, support and encourage "Research and Development" in drugs production by improving and providing funds to universities and other interested parties to aggressively intensify their efforts in other to facilitate the process.

- Offer and improve road networks and transportation for the citizens. This will help increase access to healthcare services among the population

- Easy access and availability of quality drugs, equipment, attitude of health care workers and prompt treatment encourages and increases the utilization of health care services offered and provided to the people

- Bring charity agencies to the area. This will help improve things by providing the badly needed qualified staff, medical equipment and offer the overall proper general organizational professionally needed management

- Support and provide permanent electricity solution or power generating equipment for hospitals and other health care facilities and organizations in the area

- Commend support and recognize private hospitals for their quick and prompt attention to their patients and citizens in helping to promote health and healthcare delivery in the area

- Prompt and proper government attention and interventions with specific target policies to address the negligence and inadequacies of the healthcare sector

- Above all, to stop the financial divers and spend the health care monies on health care delivery sector and projects only as directed, otherwise pay triple penalties for violation.

- Adopting the Healthcare Service Excellence Model as discussed above.

Suggestions for Future Studies

As a solution and able to survive as a system, the health care sector in Owerri must have the ability to refine, adapt and adopt to the current health care challenges and the changing environment not only in the rural areas but also the urban areas within the state of Imo and Nigeria at large. Hence, the healthcare service sector in Owerri should feature, include and implement the following additional strategies based on the findings:

- Promptness of service to improve and increase level of confidence projected and set by staff or government or agency standards;

- Improve competition among providers in the market place;

- Improve communication between providers and clients to complete explanation of treatment or service given by all levels of healthcare professionals.

- Subsidizing the high cost of drugs by the government particularly for the poor and the elderly;

- Reviewing and revising the healthcare allocation policy;

Finally, promote and improve teamwork among professionals that is currently lacking but considered important. This is essential in healthcare because when team members work together, the patient receives quality care knowing that a tree cannot make a forest by itself alone.

References

Abumere, S. I. (2002). *Rural Infrastructure and the Development Process in Rural Nigeria*. Ibahan, Nigeria: Development Policy Center.

Acho, O. (2005). Poor Healthcare System: Nigeria's Moral Indeference. Retrieved from: http://archive. is/1FAzW

Adeyemo, D. O. (2005). Local Government and Health Care Delivery in Nigeria: A Case Study. *Journal of Human Ecology, 18*(2), 149-160.

Agbo, P. (2012). Patience Jonathan's Ailment Not Detected in Nigeria. Retrieved from http://allafrica. com/stories/201209070342.html

Ajovi, S. E. (2010). The Evolution of Health Care Systems in Nigeria: Which Way Forward in the Twenty-First Century. *Nigerian Medical Journal, 51*(2), 53-65.

Akramov, T. K, (2008). Decentralization and Public Service Delivery to the Rural Poor. Washington: International Food Policy Research Institute.

Ammon, J. (2008). Dangerous Medicines: Unproven AIDS Cures and Counterfeit Antiretroviral Drugs. *East African Journal of Public Health, 5*(3), 205-210.

Andersen, R. (1968). A Behavioral Model of Families' Use of Health Services. *The Journal of Human Resources, 7*(1), 125-127.

Andersen, R. (1995). Revisiting the Behavioral Model and Access to Medical Care: Does it Matter? *Journal of Health and Social Behavior, 36*(1), 1-10.

Arodiogbu, I. L. (2005). *Introducing Social Health Insurance to Solve Problems of Poor Health in Nigeria*. Unpublished thesis, The University of Leeds, Leeds, England.

Azfar, O. (2005). Decentralization, Governance and public Services: The Impact of Institutional Arrangements. Retrieved from http://siteresources.worldbank.org/INTINDONESIA/Resources/ Decentralization/Lit_Review_IRIS.pdf

Bache, I. (1998). *The Politics of European Union Regional Policy: Multi-Level Governance or Flexible Gate keeping?* Sheffield: UACES/Sheffield Academic Press.

Bache, I., & Flinders, M. (2004). *Multi-level Governance*. Oxford: Oxford University Press.

Cockerham, W. C. (1982). *The Process of Seeking Medical Care*. Englewood Cliffs, NJ: Prentice Hall.

Cooper, D. R., & Schindler, P. S. (2008). *Business Research Methods*. New York, NY: McGraw-Hill Company.

Dare, O. (2001). Linking Health and Development in Nigeria: The Oriade Initiative. Retrieved From http://www.hsph.harvard.edu/takemi/files/2012/10/rp171.pdf.

Devarajan, S., Khemani, S., & Shah, S. (2005). Decentralization and Service Delivery. Retrieved from http://elibrary.worldbank.org/doi/pdf/10.1596/1813-9450-3603

DFID (2002). Health Insurance Workshop: Health Systems Resource Center, London. Retrieved from http://www.healthsystemsrc.org

Enthoven, A.C., & Vorhaus, C.B. (1997). A vision of quality in health care delivery. *Health Affairs*, *16*(3), 44–57.

Erhum, W. O., Babalola, O. O., & Erhun, M.O. (2001). Drug Regulation and Control in Nigeria: The Challenge of Counterfeit Drugs. *Journal of Health and Population*, *4*(2), 23-34.

Federal Republic of Nigeria; National Primary Healthcare (PHC) Development Agency, (2004). NPHCDA Annual Bulletin. Retrieved from http://cheld.org/wp-content/uploads/2012/04/Nigeria-Revised-National-Health-Policy-2004.pdf

Gaines, A. D. (1992). *Ethnopsychiatry: The cultural construction of professional and folk psychiatrics*. Albany, NY: State University of New York Press.

Garuba, H.A., Kohler, J.C., & Huisman, A.M. (2009). Transparency in Nigeria's Public Pharmaceutical Sector: Perceptions from Policy Makers. *Globalization and Health*, *5*(14), 14-27.

Gary, M. (1993). Structural Policy and Multi-level Governance in EC. Boulder, CO: Lynne Rienner Publishers.

Governor Okorocha Pledges to Transform the Health Care Sector in Imo. (2012). Retrieved from http://www.imostateblog.com/2012/09/03/governor-okorocha-pledges-to-transform-the-health-sector-in-imo/

Hasnain, Z. (2008). Devolution, Accountability, and Service Delivery: Some Insights from Pakistan. Retrieved from http://elibrary.worldbank.org/doi/pdf/10.1596/1813-9450-4610

Health Reform Foundation of Nigeria. (2007). Primary Health Care in Nigeria: 30 Years after Alma Ata. Retrieved from http://www.herfon.org/downloads/NHR2007.pdf

Healthcare. (2014). Retrieved from http://www.motherlandnigeria.com/health.html

Hooghe, L., & Gary, M. (2003). Unveiling the Central State, but How? Types of Multi-level Governance. *American Political Science Review, 97* (6), 233-43.

Hospitalized Nigerian First Lady Was Misdiagnosed By Presidential Physicians As Mystery Around Ailment Grows. (2012). Retrieved from http://saharareporters.com/news-page/hospitalized-nigeria-first-lady-was-misdiagnosed-presidential-physicians-mystery-around-ai

Ikels, C. (2002). Constructing and Deconstructing the Self: Dementia in China. *Journal of Cross-Cultural Gerontology, 17,* 233-251.

Imo State Planning and Economic development Commission, Owerri. (2005). Zero Draft "Imo Tripod Vision" State Economic Empowerment and Development Strategy (SEEDS). Retrieved from http://web.ng.undp.org/documents/SEEDS/Imo_State.pdf

Jachtenfuchs, M. (1995). Theoretical perspectives on European governance. *The European Law Journal, 1*(2), 115-133.

Janzen, J. M. (1978). *Contemporary Systems of Popular Medicine in Lower Zaire. The Quest for Therapy in Lower Zaire.* Berkeley: University of California Press.

Kamiljon, T., & Akromov, A. (2009). *Decentralization and Local Public Services in Ghana: Do Geography and Ethnic Diversity Matter?* Washington: International Food Research Institute.

Kleinman, A. (1980). *Family-Based Popular Health Care. Patients and Healers in the Context of Culture.* Berkeley, CA: University of California Press.

Kwenu: Our Culture, Our Future. (2013). Retrieved from http://archive.is/yFQfH

LaVela, S. L., Smith, B., Weaver, F. M., & Miskevics, S. A. (2004). Geographical Proximity and Health Care Utilization in Veterans with SCI &D in the USA. *Social Science and Medicine, 59,* 2387-2399.

Linden, M., Horgas, A. L, Gilberg, R., & Steinhagen-Thiessen, E. (1997). Predicting Health Care Utilization in the Very Old: The Role of Physical Health, Mental Health, Attitudinal and Social Factors. *Journal of Aging and Health, 9*(1), 3-27.

Manor, J. (1997). *The Political Economy of Democratic Decentralization.* Washington D.C: World Bank.

Megaji, B. (2010). When can Nigerians afford to buy drugs? Retrieved from http://thenationonlineng.net/web2/articles/33196/1/when-can-Nigerias-afford-buy-drugs-/Page1.html

Mourik, M. S., Cameron, A., Ewen, M., & Lang, R. O. (2010). Availability, Price and affordability of cardiovascular medicines: A comparison across 36 countries using WHO/HAI data. Retrieved from http://www.biomedcentral.com/content/pdf/1471-2261-10-25.pdf

National Population Commission of the Federal Republic of Nigeria. (2004). Nigeria Demographic and Health Survey, 2003. Retrieved from http://www.measuredhs.com/pubs/pdf/FR148/FR148.pdf

Nguyen, Q. V. (n.d.). Decentralization and Local Governance on Public Services Delivery: The cases of Daknong and Hau-giang province in Vietnam. Retrieved from http://papers.ssrn.com/sol3/cf_dev/AbsByAuth.cfm?per_id=989308

Nigeria: Health Sector Management Chaotic, Says Expert. (2005). Retrieved from http://allafrica.com/stories/200502110203.html

Nigeria Ranked Second Most Corrupt Country. (n.d.). Retrieved from http://www.onlinenigeria.com/adprint.asp?blurb=78

Ogundipe, S., (2010). Proposed Drug Ban Offers Nigerians No Safety Net. Retrieved from http://www.vanguardngr.com/2010/04/proposed-drug-ban-offers-nigerians-no-safety-net/

Oguzor, N. (2011). A Spatial Analysis of Infrastructure and Social Services in Rural Nigeria: Implications for Public service. Retrieved from http://www.geotropico.org/NS_5_1_Oguzor.pdf

Ojeifo, M. O. (2008). Problems of Effective Primary Healthcare Delivery in Owan East and Owan West Local Government Areas of Edo State, Nigeria. *Journal of Social Science 16*(1), 69–77.

Okali, D. U., Okpara, E. E., & Olawole, J, (2001). The Case of Aba and its Region, South East Nigeria. Retrieved from http://pubs.iied.org/9117IIED.html

Okhamefe, A. O. (2006). From Rubbish to Riches, Trash to Treasure. Retrieved from http://www.uniben.edu/sites/default/files/inaugural_lectures/ProfOkhamafe1.pdf

Okorochas, O. (2012). The Year 2012 Budget. Retrieved from http://reclaimnaija.net/Budgets/state/IMO-STATE-GOVERNMENT-BUDGET-SPEECH-2012.pdf

Olayiwola, L. M., & Adeleye, O. A. (2005). Rural Infrastructural Development in Nigeria between 1960 –1990: Problems and Challenges. *Journal of Social Science, 11*(2), 91-96.

Onimode, B. (1988). *A Political Economy of African Crisis*. New Jersey: Zed Books.

Onokerhoraye, A. G. (1999). Access and Utilization of Modern Health Care Facilities in the Petroleum-Producing Region of Nigeria: The Case of Bayelsa State. Retrieved from http://hsph.andplus.com/takemi/files/2012/10/rp162.pdf.

Orabuchi, A. (2005). Poor Healthcare System: Nigeria's Moral Indifference. Retrieved from http://archive.is/1FAzW

Peters, B. G., & Pierre, J. (2001). Developments in Intergovernmental Relations: Towards Multi-Level Governance. *Policy and Politics, 29*(2), 131-135.

Predeeep, H. U. S. (2011). Challenges of Local Government Service Delivery: A Case Study of Matara Municipal Council. Retrieved from http://lgbd.org/cms_lg-publication-other-countries-_50_0

Rahman, H. M. and Khan, M. M, (1997). Decentralization and Access: Theoretical Framework and Bangladesh Experience. *Asian Profile, 25*(6), 513-526.

Rebhan, D. P. (n.d.). Health Care Utilization: Understanding and Applying Theories and Models of Health Care Seeking Behavior. Case Western University.

Reichheld, F. F. (2003). The One Number you Need to Know. Retrieved from http://hbr.org/2003/12/the-one-number-you-need-to-grow/

Robertson, J. (2003). Sending in the SWOT team. Retrieved from http://www.pks.org/operations/helpful/get_file.php?f=Is_Your_Chapter_Ready_to_SWOT_the_Competition.PDF

Rosenstock, I. M., Strecher, V. J., & Becker, M. H. (1994). *The Health Belief Model and HIV Risk Behavior Change.* US: Springer.

Satmetrix Systems, Inc. (2007). The Power Behind a Single Number: A White Paper. Retrieved from http://www.ccsdelivered.com/whitepapers/Net%20Promoter%20-%20The%20Power%20Behind%20A%20Single%20Number.pdf

Scot, H. R. (2002). Decentralization: Does it Deliver Good Governance and Improved Service? The Experience of Uganda. Coventary University: African Studies Center.

Social Infrastructure. (n.d.). Retrieved from http://www.onlinenigeria.com/links/LinksReadPrint.asp?blurb=271

Stubbs, P. (2005). Stretching Concepts Too Far? Multi-Level Governance, Policy Transfer and the Politics of Scale in South Eastern Europe. *Southeast European Politics Online, 6*(2), 66-88.

Taylor, S., & Fields, D. (Eds.). (2003). *Approaches to Health, Illness, and Health Care.* Oxford: Blackwell Publishing

Transparency Int'l Ranks Nigeria 35th Most Corrupt. (2012). Retrieved from http://www.thenigerianvoice.com/nvnews/102810/1/transparency-intl-ranks-nigeria-35th-most-corrupt-.html

Udenwa, T. (2010). Why Drugs are Expensive in Nigeria. Retrieved from http://www.nigerianbestforum.com/blog/why-drugs-are-expensive-nigeria-2/

United Nations Development Program. (1999). Decentralization: A Sampling Of Definitions. Retrieved from http://web.undp.org/evaluation/documents/decentralization_working_report.PDF

United Nations Department of Economic and Social Affairs. (2009). World Population Ageing 2009 Report. Retrieved from http://www.un.org/esa/population/publications/WPA2009/WPA2009_WorkingPaper.pdf

United Nations, Department of Economic and Social Affairs. (2007). World Population Ageing 2007 Report. Retrieved from http://www.un.org/en/development/desa/population/publications/pdf/ageing/WorldPopulationAgeingReport2007.pdf

United Nations Economic Commission for Africa. (2012). Africa's Economic Growth has not Created Enough Jobs for Youth, Experts Say. Retrieved from http://www1.uneca.org/TabId/3018/Default.aspx?ArticleId=2241

Uwadi, K. (2001). Why Owerri is Now Rated as Nigeria's Dirtiest City. Retrieved from http://www.igbofocus.co.uk/html/imo_state.html

Wolinsky, F. D. (1988). Seeking and using health services. In Wolinsky, F. D. (Ed.), *The Sociology of Health, Principles Practitioners and Issues* (pp. 117-144). Belmont, CA : Wadsworth Publishing Company.

World Bank (n.d.). World development indicators: Nigeria. Retrieved from http://data.worldbank.org/country/nigeria

World Bank. (2000). The World Development Report 1999-2000: Entering the 21st Century. Retrieved from http://wdronline.worldbank.org//worldbank/bookpdfdownload/21

World Bank. (2003). World Development Report 2004: Making Services Work For Poor People. Retrieved from http://web.worldbank.org/WBSITE/EXTERNAL/EXTDEC/EXTRESEARCH/EXTWDRS/0,,contentMDK:23062333~pagePK:478093~piPK:477627~theSitePK:477624,00.html

World Bank. (2005). Meeting the Challenge of Africa's Development. Retrieved from http://siteresources.worldbank.org/INTAFRICA/Resources/aap_final.pdf

World Bank. (2007). India - Rural Governments and Service Delivery: Volume 1, Executive Summary. Retrieved from https://openknowledge.worldbank.org/handle/10986/8007

World Health Organization. (n.d.). WHO Statistical Information System. Health Statistics for Nigeria. Retrieved from http://www.who.int/gho/en/

World Health Organization. (1999). The World Health Report 1999—Making a Difference. Retrieved from http://www.who.int/whr/1999/en/

World Health Organization. (2000). The World Health Report 2000. Retrieved from http://www.who.int/whr/2000/en/

World Health Organization. (2010). Trends in Maternal Mortality: 1990 – 2010. Retrieved from http://www.nitpn.com/pdf%20docs/soplanning.pdf

Young, J.C. (1981). *Medical Choice in a Mexican Village.* New Brunswick, N.J.: Rutgers University Press.

Young, J.C., & Garro-Young, L. (1982). Variations in the Choice of Treatment in Two Mexican Communities. *Social Science and Medicine, 16*(16), 1453–1465.

Appendix A: Cover Letter

Dear Respondent,

As a candidate for the doctoral degree at California InterContinental University, I am conducting a research project concerning the delivery of health care services in Owerri and in the State of Imo. I am a healthcare professional and a native of Owerri and my research is driven by my commitment to help improve healthcare in Nigeria.

This enclosed survey questionnaire is used to seek your opinion on what you would like to see happen to improve health care services in Owerri and the State as a whole.

I would appreciate it if you could complete the questionnaire in its entirety. Keep in mind that this is your government and you have the power and authority to voice your opinion, say and tell what you want the government to do for you for your own welfare. Information you provide will be used to persuade decision makers to resolve issues and improve the quality of health care services. This questionnaire is designed to maintain your anonymity. This means that no one will know your name or who you are. Opinions and concerns that you express in this questionnaire will be organized into a cohesive and meaningful set of recommendations that I will forward to decision makers and to you upon the successful completion of this research study.

Thank you in advance for your assistance and contribution in this academic inquiry. Please feel free to contact me at any time.

Sincerely Yours,

Mr. Lambert Nwachukwu

RN Northeast Georgia Medical Center,

743 Spring Street, Gainesville, GA. 30501

Email: adachidit@att.net

California InterContinental University, Diamond Bar, California, USA.

Appendix B: Interview Questions for Civil Servants

PART 1 - Personal Information

1.1 Please kindly indicate your age:

18-24

25-30

31-35

36-40

41-45

46-50

51-55

56-60

61-65

66+

1.2 What gender are you?

Male Female

1.3 Do you live alone?

Yes No

1.4

A) Please indicate your marital status.

Married Divorced Single

B) Do you have children?

Yes No

C) If yes above, how many children do you have?

1.5a Are you a student?

Yes No

1.5b What is your level of education? Choose one:

A) Elementary School graduate

B) Secondary School graduate

C) Did not Graduate Secondary school

D) University Graduate

E) Masters' Degree

F) Doctorate Degree

1.6 If you were to evaluate your health, what would you say? P/s briefly describe or explain below.

1.7

A) Where in Imo State do you live?

B) What is the name of your Local Government Area?

1.8 How often do you go for your medical checkup in a year? . . . . . .

1.9 Which hospital do you use or go to?

1.10 A) Which medical facility do you like most? Choose one:

A) Federal Medical Center (FMC)

B) Local Government Center

C) Patented Chemist

D) Traditional Treatment

E) Other

B) Why do you like this method of treatment or go to this place?

1.11 How many hospitals are in your local government?

1.12 Do you use traditional medicine (as an alternative) in meeting your health care needs?

1.14 How effective is the use of traditional medicine in meeting your health care service needs?

1.15 How far is the hospital from your house or home?

1.16 Do you have your own primary (personal) care doctor?

Yes No

1.17 How far do you live from your doctor?

1.18

A) How long have you known your doctor?

B) How often do you see him for medical reasons?

1.19 What kind of doctor is s/he? Choose one:

A) Internal Medicine

B) Neuro-Surgeon

C) Cardiologist

D) Ortho-Doctor

E) General Practice

F) Don't know

1.20 How satisfied are you with your doctor? Choose one:

A) Very satisfied

B) Satisfied

C) Average

D) Unsatisfied

1.2 What gender are you?

Male Female

1.3 Do you live alone?

Yes No

1.4 A Please indicate your marital status?

Married Divorced Single

B) Do you have children?

Yes No

C) If yes above, how many children do you have?

1.5a Are you a student?

Yes No

1.5b What is your level of education? Choose one:

A) Elementary School graduate

B) Secondary School graduate

C) Did not Graduate Secondary School

D) University Graduate

E) Masters' Degree

F) Doctorate Degree

1.6 If you were to evaluate your health, what would you say? P/s briefly describe or explain below.

1.7 A) Where in Imo State do you live?

B) What is the name of your Local Government Area?

1.8 How often do you go for your medical checkup in a year?

1.9 Which hospital do you use or go to?

1.10 A) Which medical facility do you like most? Choose one:

A) Federal Medical Center (FMC)

B) Local Government Center

C) Patented Chemist

D) Traditional treatment

E) Other

B) Why do you like this method of treatment or go to this place?

1.11 How many hospitals are in your local government?

1.12 Do you use traditional medicine (as an alternative) in meeting your health care needs?

1.14 How effective is the use of traditional medicine in meeting your health care service needs?

1.15 How far is the hospital from your house or home?

1.16 Do you have your own primary (personal) care doctor?

Yes No

1.17 How far do you live from your doctor?

1.18 A) How long have you known your doctor?

B) How often do you see him for medical reasons?

1.19 What kind of doctor is s/he? Choose one:

A) Internal Medicine

B) Neuro-Surgeon

C) Cardiologist

D) Ortho-Doctor

E) General Practice

F) Don't know

1.20 How satisfied are you with your doctor? Choose one:

A) Very satisfied

B) Satisfied

C) Average

D) Unsatisfied

1.21.1 How do you go to your doctor for appointments?

1.21.2 Does the government provide you with transportation?

Yes No

1.22 If you use or spend your own money for transportation, does the government refund you or pay you back your money?

Yes No

1.23 What prevents you from seeing your doctor more often?

1.24 Why did you go to the doctor the last time?

1.25 What was the diagnosis of your last visit?

1.26 Are you worried about the standard of health care service delivery in Owerri?

Yes No

1.27 What do you see as the health care needs of the population in Owerri?

1.28 What changes about health care services delivery would you like to see in Owerri?

1.29 What are the key health care challenges confronting health care organizations in Owerri?

1.30 Do you think there is a need for foreign charities to promote and provide health care services in Owerri?

1.31 How important to you is free health care service in Owerri? Choose one:

A) Very important

B) Important

C) Unimportant

1.32 Would you like to see health care insurance coverage implemented in Owerri City?

Yes No

If yes, explain

If no, explain .

1.33 Would you like to pay a little money to help the government cover the citizens' of Owerri for improved health care service?

Yes No

If yes above, how much contribution out of your pay check are you willing to make? Choose one.

A) 1-5 %

B) 6 - 10%

C) 11 - 15%

D) 16 - 20%

E) 21 - 25%

F) 26+ %

PART 2 - Employment

2.0 Are you currently employed?

Yes No

2.1 If yes, which ministry do you work for?

2.2 Do you work for a private company?

Yes No

2.3 Are you a management staff?

Yes No

2.4 How long have you worked for this ministry?

How long have worked for this private company?

2.5 How much do you make a month?. Choose one:

A) Less than 20,000

B) 21,000 t0 30,000

C) 31,000 to 40,000

D) 41,000 to 50,000

E) 51,000 to 60,000

F) 61,000 to 70,000

G) 71,000 to 80,000

H) 81,000 to 90,000

I) 91,000 to 100,000

J) 101,000+

2.6 How much do you spend on medical expenses each month?

2.7 Do you have medical insurance?

Yes No

2.8 A) Does your job pay or cover your medical expenses?

Yes No

B) Does your job cover your medical insurance?

Yes No

2.9 If yes above, how much does your employer pay a month toward your health insurance?

2.10 Is your insurance coverage individual or family?

A) Individual B) Family

2.11 How much does your employer pay or contribute for your health insurance each month?

2.12 Does your employer refund you out pocket medical expenses monthly?

2.13 How much medical expenses does your employer pay back or refund you each month?

PART 3—State Questions

3.1) How is health care service delivered in Owerri?

3.2 A) Are you worried about the health care service delivery system in Owerri?

Yes No

B) If your answer is "Yes" above Why?

C) if your answer above is "No" Why not?

3.3 Are you worried about the health care services delivery system in

Imo State?

Yes No

If your answer is "Yes" Why?

If your answer is "No" Why not?

3.4 What do think the government should do to improve health care service in Imo State?

3.5 How important to you is free health care service in Imo State?

Choose one:

A) Very important

B) Important

C) Unimportant

3.6 Would you like to see health care insurance coverage implemented in

Imo State?

Yes No

3.7 Would you like to pay a little money to help the government cover the citizens' of Imo State for improved

health care service?

Yes No

If yes above, how much contribution out of your paycheck are you willing to make? Chose one:

A) 1-5 %

B) 6 - 10%

C) 11 - 15%

D) 16 - 20%

E) 21 - 25%

F) 26+%

3.8 Are you worried about the standard of health care service delivery in Imo State?

Yes No

If "yes" Why?

3.9 What do you see as the health care service needs of the population in Imo State?

3.10 What changes about health care services delivery would you like to see in Imo State?

3.11 What are the key health care challenges confronting health care organizations in Imo State?

3.12 Do you think there is a need for foreign charities to promote and provide health care services in Imo State?

Yes No

If your answer is "Yes", explain below.

If no, explain.

Part 4—Interview Questionnaire for Managers

Name: . . .

Position:

1. What is your role/function at the Council/Ministry of Health Owerri?

2. Do you provide health services to the public? If yes, what health services?

3. How many years have you been in your current post?

4. What is your education background?

5. Do service seekers give their full support to you addressing their needs? Yes /No.

If no, why the opposition?

6. Did service seekers' behavior have any influence to consider service delivery? If yes, how do they try to influence it (the process)?

7. (a) Do you have sufficient staff in facility, hospital, or organization to take care of your clients or service seekers? Yes or No.

(b) If no, why not?

8. Do you have sufficient physical resources in the discharge of your responsibility? Yes / No (please give reasons for your answer)

a) Vehicles

b) Communication Facilities (Telephone, Internet and Fax)

c) Computers

d) Typewriters

9. (a) Did you experience/observe a change in the service delivery strategy of the Council /Ministry after 2005?

(b) If not why not and if yes what did you experience/observed?

(c) And which of these successes or appropriateness addressed the problems of service delivery?

10. In your opinion, what are the different problems that are related to or with the challenges that affect the better health service delivery of the Council/ Ministry in Owerri?

11. Do you have any suggestions to how the Council/ Ministry can overcome its challenges?

Part 5—Interview Questionnaire on Civil Society Leaders

Name:

Organization:

Position:

1. What is your organization's role in delivering health services in Owerri?

2. How your' organization make a link between service provider and service seekers?

3 a) Do you give full support to the Council/Ministry for delivering health services? Yes / No.

b) If no, why the opposition?

4. a) Did you experience/observe a change in the service delivery strategy of the Council or Ministry after 2005?

b) If not why not and if yes what did you experience/observed?

c) And which of these successes is being addressed the problems of service delivery?

5 a) Are you satisfied with the current standards/quality of service delivery in Owerri?

b) If yes, why? And if not, why not?

6) In your opinion, what are the different problems relating to the challenges affecting better healthcare service delivery by the council in Owerri/Imo State?

7) Do you have any suggestions to how the Council/Ministry can overcome these challenges or solving its problems?

The city is located in the heart of Igbo Land or Southeastern Nigeria, and its motto is *Heartland*. Rich in history and tradition, and in spite of a tumultuous past as the capital of the Republic of Biafra during the 1960s, the city is considered to be the entertainment capital of present-day Nigeria, home of excellent academic institutions and healthcare centers, a bustling economy, as well the home of the annual pageant of Miss Heartland.

Mr. Rochas Anayo Okorocha, the current Owelle or Governor of the state of Imo, is an elected public official who, according to published reports is fully committed to implementing programs, projects and initiates to improving health care conditions in Owerri and the whole state

The Federal Medical Center of Owerri is a potential participant in this research project.

The Community Health Center in Owerri is a potential participant in this research project.

Imo State University is a potential participant in this research project.

The Federal University of Technology in Owerri is a potential participant in the research project.

Alvan Ikoku College of Education in Owerri is a potential participant in the research project.

Printed in the United States
By Bookmasters